PRAISE FOR TELL MY SONS

"Mark Weber's book, *Tell My Sons...*, is a poignant illustration of what being a hero is all about. Heroes exemplify invincible courage, character, and perseverance in times of insurmountable odds. Mark embodies these attributes. *Tell My Sons...* will empower the reader with profound lessons of living life with hope and determination!"

—JOHN ELWAY, PRO FOOTBALL HALL OF FAME QUARTERBACK AND TWO-TIME SUPER BOWL CHAMPION OF THE DENVER BRONCOS

"Mark Weber is a modern-day soldier-statesman who has given us a blueprint for how to build character—an indispensable quality for transformative and sustainable leadership."

—TIM PAWLENTY, FORMER GOVERNOR OF MINNESOTA AND REPUBLICAN PRESIDENTIAL CANDIDATE

"A powerful testimony of compassion, conviction, and persistence. Mark is an incredibly talented communicator who has provided us all with an intimate and intellectually gripping perspective on life. He pulls no punches—with his sons, with us, or with himself. With humility and a gift for bridging sobering topics, *Tell My Sons...* will inspire you to want to be a better human being."

—CATHY L. GREENBERG, PHD, CO-AUTHOR OF THE *NEW YORK TIMES*-BESTSELLER, *WHAT HAPPY WORKING MOTHERS KNOW* AND *WHAT HAPPY WOMEN KNOW*

"You three boys, along with your father, Mark, have given-names that belonged to men who are surely in God's 'Hall of Fame of Faith.' . . . None of us knows the challenges we will face, but we know that to meet those challenges God has a great reservoir of mental, physical, and moral strength for each of us. . . . Your dad has given you an unadorned look at his courageous use of those reservoirs in meeting the challenges for him and your family. It will surely help you in meeting your own challenges."

—GENERAL JOHN W. VESSEY, JR., US ARMY (RET),
10TH CHAIRMAN OF THE JOINT CHIEFS OF STAFF

"Mark Weber's *Tell My Sons...* should be entitled *Tell Us All.* This poignant, passionate, and very personal work will deeply move you. Yes it's a story for Mark's sons, but it is much more. Here is one man's life story, a soldier's story, that has the wisdom of a life well lived. It's a great legacy for his sons, but it's a great legacy for our sons and daughters as well."

—GENERAL RICHARD MYERS, US AIR FORCE (RET),
15TH CHAIRMAN OF THE JOINT CHIEFS OF STAFF

"The Webers have served the US Army and our nation with great distinction, and their recent battle with cancer is no exception. Mark has soldiered on, pouring his great courage, dogged determination, and unflinching humor into the most painful gift a father can give. He has written answers to questions that have yet to be asked, turning personal lessons into a powerful legacy. *Tell My Sons...* will leave an indelible mark on the hearts of all who read it. Lynne and I are honored to have served with the Weber family; we are inspired by their story, which will continue to inspire for generations to come."

—GENERAL PETER PACE, US MARINE CORPS (RET),
16TH CHAIRMAN OF THE JOINT CHIEFS OF STAFF

"The ancients admired most the man who could face mortality and still tell a great story. They would surely admire Mark Weber. Here you'll find the truest heroism."

—JAY HEINRICHS, AUTHOR OF *THANK YOU FOR ARGUING*

"Mark and Kristin Weber's courage along their journey of life exemplify the Outward Bound values, 'To serve, to strive, and not to yield.' Thanks to this book, his sons won't be the only ones who benefit from this wonderful gift of mentorship and empowerment."

—LEE SKOLD, CHAIRMAN OF THE BOARD, OUTWARD BOUND USA

"Mark has crafted a moving account of pain and suffering turned into joy and wisdom. Through all the hardships and battles, he displays the fighting spirit of a warrior, the steady compassion of a leader, and the unconditional love of a father and husband. His life and his words are an inspiration to me, and they will be an inspiration to you."

—ERIC GREITENS, *NEW YORK TIMES*-BESTSELLING AUTHOR OF *THE HEART AND THE FIST: THE EDUCATION OF A HUMANITARIAN, THE MAKING OF A NAVY SEAL*

"*Tell My Sons...* is an inspiring work of great and earthy humanity, full of precious models of wisdom and honest love. Mark's story reveals the importance of exercising reflective curiosity and empathic imagination in serving with grace, care, and good humor. He has taught me about how honest human beings respond to a life that they allow themselves to love."

—DR. RONALD HEIFETZ, FOUNDING DIRECTOR, CENTER FOR PUBLIC LEADERSHIP AT HARVARD UNIVERSITY, AND AUTHOR OF *LEADERSHIP WITHOUT EASY ANSWERS*

"I've been around Mark Weber a lot in some incredibly difficult circumstances, and it was not only what he got done, but how he got it done. . . . It's not a bad thing when you come across someone who can influence you so profoundly, whether you're a Private First Class or the Chairman of the Joint Chiefs of Staff of the United States of America. . . . He's one of the finest leaders I've met in my thirty-eight years of service."

—General Martin E. Dempsey, US Army,
18th Chairman of the Joint Chiefs of Staff

"You've been fighting a courageous personal battle since I almost had you on a plane to Afghanistan two years ago, and I truly have been inspired by your bravery and grit."

—General David H. Petraeus, US Army (Ret),
Director of the Central Intelligence Agency

TELL MY SONS...

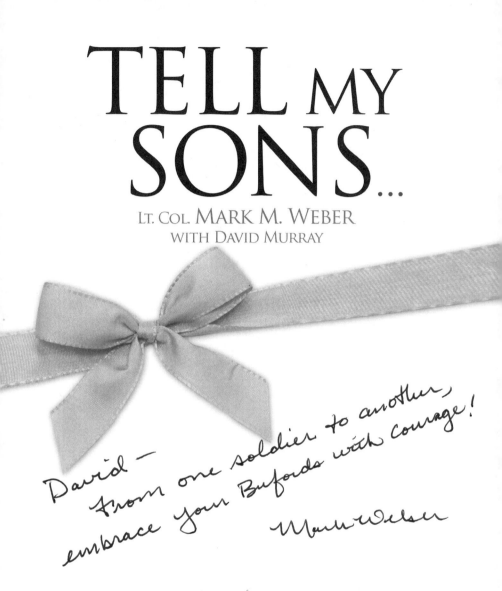

TELL MY SONS...

Lt. Col. MARK M. WEBER
WITH DAVID MURRAY

David —
From one soldier to another,
embrace your Bufords with courage!

Mark Weber

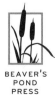

BEAVER'S
POND
PRESS

With David Murray

ISBN 13: 978-1-59298-570-8

Library of Congress Catalog Number: 2012920674

Printed in the United States of America

First Printing: 2013

17 16 15 14 13   5 4 3 2 1

Author photo by Allison Lea Photography, July 2010.
Cover photo and compass were provided by Mark and Kristin Weber.
Cover and interior design by James Monroe Design, LLC.

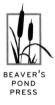

BEAVER'S
POND
PRESS

Beaver's Pond Press, Inc.
7108 Ohms Lane
Edina, MN 55439–2129
(952) 829-8818
www.BeaversPondPress.com

To order, visit www.BeaversPondBooks.com
or call (800) 901-3480. Reseller discounts available.

Please visit: TellMySons.com

For Matthew, Joshua, and Noah

Kristin and I are going to use fifty percent of the proceeds from this book to help other parents' sons and daughters overcome their hardships so they may live, as I hope my sons will, rich and productive and loving lives.

CONTENTS

Each of these titles comes from a farewell speech
General Douglas MacArthur delivered in 1962 to the
Corps of Cadets at the US Army Military Academy
at West Point.

FOREWORD

We all eventually reach the end of our march. For some of us, the route is long. For others, the path is short. But it's not the length of the journey that matters as much as the steps we take.

If you discovered disease was about to cut your life short, no one could rightfully judge you for dropping out of line. But for those who refuse to let an incurable illness keep them from doing their duty, for those who keep fighting, for those who live life vigorously and joyfully to the very end, we have names for those people. We call them heroes.

I had the pleasure of working with Mark during a USO tour he helped organize for the chairman of the Joint Chiefs of Staff in 2004. At the time, he inspired me in the same way all military personnel do. Everyone who serves their country deserves respect for their personal sacrifice, and they sure get mine. But after learning of his battle with cancer, my respect for Mark grew exponentially.

If war is hell, as they say, then fighting an incurable disease is something altogether worse.

Soldiers can survive wars. Cancer victims in stage IV aren't usually so fortunate. As the fight continues, the odds dwindle. That can either be a cause for isolation or an opportunity to send a powerful message with whatever life one has left to live. Mark Weber chose the latter. Instead of shutting down, Mark got to work. He collected his thoughts and stories for his sons, and we're fortunate he's left them behind for us all to read.

Lt. Col. Weber marched with purpose, humor, dignity, and grace. This book is about what drove him. It's a look at who he was, what he believed, and what awaits his sons in their own lives. Reading it might help you advance through this world, too.

May he light the way.

—Robin Williams

PREFACE

Dear Matthew, Joshua, and Noah–

I wrote a book for you. I started writing it long before any of you were born, and even before I met your mom, but it was always written for you.

When I was twelve years old, my grandma Weber died of a sudden heart attack. As we helped Grandpa go through her things, we came across a letter he wrote to her in August 1944. His work kept them separated, and he was writing to tell her about his job, the weather—no mention of the world war raging across the sea— and how "it seems like it has been a year here without you." He was playful. He drew several doodles in the margins, one of which was a man sticking out his tongue. He closed the note by telling her how much he enjoyed the roast and the cake she made for him, and then he drew two birds—one for each of his sons at the time.

The faded letter looked and felt like an ancient treasure, but what impressed me most was that I had never heard Grandpa talk or act that sweet. He didn't even remember writing it and said it didn't sound like him at all. That bugged me. I wanted to know more about Grandma. And I sure wouldn't want to forget what it was like to write a letter like that.

As I grew older, I found that all my grandparents were short on details. Of course, they had stories, but not always the details I wanted to know about. They couldn't remember young emotions or reasoning, and they wouldn't talk about their biggest mistakes or regrets. The questions I had didn't match the answers they were willing or able to give.

I imagined someday I would have grandkids (yes, grandkids) who might be just as interested in me as I was in my grandparents. And so I started writing a journal, and I kept it brutally honest. Looking back, there's a lot of stuff I'm really not proud of, but I figure maybe those ugly things reflect my growth through the years. This book comes from that journal.

Of course, I imagined one day sharing these stories in person, but now I'm dying, and I realize I might not even get to share it with you boys, let alone with any grandkids.

If attitude alone determined survival, I would live another fifty years. Unfortunately, our bodies get a vote, and my forty-year-old frame is giving out way sooner than it should. Despite some breathtaking treatments, I still have cancer, I can't have any more surgeries, and the chemo is failing. I may look invincible in my army uniform or while cutting down trees with a feeding machine strapped over my shoulder, but to suggest that I'm not dying is just dishonest.

So I started thinking about ways to tell you my stories.

There's an eighteen-year-old boy inside of me who sees the three of you quickly approaching the age when I started really thinking about life. That boy stood out on a parade field twenty-three years ago as a day-four enlisted soldier in the army and listened while an unseen narrator passionately recited an adaptation of General Douglas MacArthur's famous 1962 speech to the cadets of West Point. The words and the accompanying music pulled at the hair on my arms and neck, and I felt tears roll down my cheeks. For the first time—and forever after—I understood life was much bigger than the things that were happening around me.

I committed the speech to memory and have recited it with the same passion during countless retirement ceremonies and military holidays over the past twenty years. You three were all just babies when the army recognized me as one of the best company grade officers of the 30,000-plus in the army. The honor? The General MacArthur Leadership Award.

The truth is, I'm not a big fan of Douglas MacArthur and never have been. I attended a military high school and have been in an army uniform since age fourteen, so I knew who MacArthur was when I first heard his words. He always seemed more movie character than actual man, and it struck me then that if you want to be a real-life man, you have to learn from real-life men.

But his speech to those young men is about being a real man. It's about life as a struggle and our need to embrace it, about the contradictions and complexity and confusion, about the courage and search for wisdom required to get through it all, and about coming to it all as honestly as a man can reasonably do.

So when it came time to share with you what I've learned about life, I knew I had to draw on that speech just one more time—with the three of you as my aspiring young "cadets," and each chapter framed in a moral from that speech.

Matthew, when you were twelve, I tried to offer you some advice after a brief discussion on some mundane subject, and you interrupted me. "Dad," you said with an elevated tone to get my attention, "I'll figure it out." You were right then, and you're still right. You had asked the question, gained some context, and then set out on your own course. With such understanding, I have faith that the three of you will indeed figure it out.

And so these pages reflect observations and perspective rather than advice or instruction. Though I'll speak with my usual conviction and passion, I know I gained those attributes over a long period of time and in the same manner Matthew expressed. My stories are not examples of the way to live your life; my stories are just examples of an infinite number of paths.

Which one should you take?

With the help of many other people you'll meet in your life—you'll figure it out.

Along the way, I hope you'll consult these pages as often and as casually as you would if I were still here and you could pick up the phone. I hope you'll ask this book different questions at different times in your lives. And I hope you'll find answers or perspective to match.

I hate writing this letter, but I would hate not writing it even more. Nothing can replace the long talks I hoped to have while fishing or driving to some far-off adventure with you, just as I got to do with my dad. But, thankfully, I've been blessed with enough time to pass along the most compelling experiences of my life. As sad as the reasons are for writing any of this, let's see if we can squeeze some joy out of it before I have to leave.

Love,
Dad

INTRODUCTION

. . . To be strong enough to know when
you are weak, brave enough to face yourself
when you are afraid.

June 2010

It's a Wednesday afternoon, and General David Petraeus has
just assumed command of all operations in Afghanistan following a very public dismissal of General Stanley McChrystal. The
last time a president sacked a general for poor conduct was when
Harry Truman fired General Douglas MacArthur over disagreement on war strategy in Korea.

Most of the senior army leaders in the Minnesota National
Guard knew Petraeus had selected me for an assignment to Iraq in
2005–2006, when I was a major and still in the US Regular Army.
Many also knew I had maintained a loose relationship with him
since then and that he had recently accepted a personal invitation to
come visit Minnesota. My comrades half-joked I would get a call.

There was no call from Petraeus, but there was an e-mail, and in it he proposed I join his team in Afghanistan on a special mission with the most senior levels of the Afghan parliament.

Petraeus reached out to one of his two subordinate general officers, and twelve hours later, I received an unexpected call on my cell phone while sitting in morning rush hour traffic on I-35E.

"Mark, this is Lieutenant General Caldwell"—that's three stars—"calling from Afghanistan . . . Do you have time to talk?"

We had never met, but he spoke in a tone and language that experience taught me was reserved for personal staff and a mature relationship. He told me an endorsement from Petraeus was as good as it got, "so let's get to it."

He asked what I had done to earn such high praise and how I had maintained such a long-term relationship with senior Iraqi leaders—specifically, General Babakir Zibari, the Iraqi chief of defense, to whom I was assigned during my deployment. My explanation sounded modest, but it was the truth—lots of energy, simple social graces, and learning Kurdish, the Iraqi general's native language. Caldwell didn't seem to believe it was that simple but commented, "Well, we want and need *that* kind of talent."

I lay in bed that night, staring at the ceiling, my mind cluttered with mixed emotions. I'd have to leave you all immediately for a yearlong absence in a war zone, which made me sad and anxious. On the other hand, combat is why soldiers exist, it had been five years since I last deployed, and this kind of assignment and professional affirmation was as good as it got for a soldier of *any* rank.

I wondered whether the request would ruffle feathers with Minnesota's army leadership, who would have to replace me, knowing there *were* other army officers qualified for such an assignment. The anxiety was misplaced. Major General Larry Shellito, the adjutant general of Minnesota, shared Caldwell's e-mail with me when it arrived:

Mark excelled as the Military Assistant to the Iraqi Chief of Defense during his last tour in Iraq. Based on his past experience and proven stellar performance, would like to offer him the opportunity to contribute as the Military Assistant to the incoming Afghan Minister of the Interior, Bismillah Mohammadi. His unique skill set and proven ability to navigate the nuances/ambiguities of this very non-standard mission would be an invaluable addition to the team here. We are entering a critical time in the Ministries and Mark could bring a tremendous vantage point . . . General Petraeus and I have spoken about Mark and if you are in agreement, would really like to bring him onboard . . . Letting Mark go would cause your team to go without, but if you are able to make this work we would be grateful.

General Shellito immediately approved the courtesy request. In fact, within a week, he approved my immediate promotion to lieutenant colonel.

At home, there was a peace and serenity unusual for a deployment. Kristin (she may be Mom to you, but she'll be Kristin to me throughout this story) accepted the news with quiet resolve. She wasn't excited about it, but she was completely unshaken. She was used to disruptive military life, but this time—for the first time in my career—she was right where she wanted to be during a deployment.

She was home *in Minnesota.*

Her sister and parents lived two and fifteen miles away, respectively. Both of our families were within an hour's drive. She also knew that when I returned from the deployment, she wouldn't need to worry about being moved to a new assignment and a new home, as we had after previous deployments.

I was being delivered to a promotion and a dream assignment with implications on an international scale. Kristin was as content as she had ever been with the chaos that is army life. You boys were getting to know your extended family in ways you never could before.

It might have been the happiest moment of my life.

The only remaining hurdle was self-imposed. Though already medically cleared to deploy, I wanted a more thorough look. For three years, I had been diagnosed with a bleeding ulcer, but this was no ordinary ulcer. Twice I had experienced a massive hemorrhage in my small intestine, and the first one nearly killed me.

Perhaps you remember eating Thanksgiving dinner without me in 2007 while I was in the hospital seven states away, or when my chair sat empty just after Matthew's thirteenth birthday in 2009 while I was in the hospital. The ulcer slowly bled over the next eighteen months.

History told me I was due for another episode. It didn't take much imagination to guess how things would end up if I hemorrhaged during a mission to some remote corner of Afghanistan.

As alarming as these incidents sound, I was tempted to blow them off. Two civilian gastrointestinal specialists said I had a non-life-threatening condition thousands of people learn to live with. Each one dismissed the idea that the trouble could be anything other than an ulcer, and I had no reason to doubt them. I had just moved about sixteen yards of mulch into our backyard (yes, with your help, Matthew), and I was running two miles three times a week. I did feel tired, but it didn't seem abnormal. I was convinced I had an undiagnosed bacterial infection or a small aneurism near the intestinal wall.

It took a week to see my third GI specialist in as many years—Dr. Jake Matlock. He said the ulcer diagnoses from past doctors weren't exactly wrong, but my symptoms demanded a closer look with the use of an endoscopy (a lighted scope lowered down the throat and into the stomach). I'd had this procedure twice before, so I knew what to expect.

After the procedure, Dr. Matlock came into my room wearing a bit of a poker face. He said he had found a fist-size lesion in my duodenum (small intestine just past the stomach). It was about ten times bigger than the ulcer's description from the year prior. He also told me normal stores of iron in the blood run from 100 to 300. Mine were at two.

I didn't need any translation on those numbers, but I still didn't think I had anything a blood transfusion, antibiotics, and some cauterization wouldn't fix. He ordered a CT scan.

Kristin and I returned the next day to discuss the results of the scan. We nervously chatted with each other as we waited. My mind was mostly elsewhere: my deployment clock was ticking loudly in my head, and I was focused on the new Afghan minister.

Dr. Matlock entered the room and quickly took a seat. His face was expressionless, and he wasted no time delivering his message. He spoke with a soft and compassionate voice: "Mark, I'm afraid the news is bad . . . really bad. The 'ulcer' is not an ulcer. You have cancer."

The words seemed to come out of his mouth in slow motion. The scene didn't seem real. It was more like the set of a movie, with me playing a character. I tried to discount the significance of the news, but the CT images wouldn't let me.

"This entire area here, where the stomach connects to the intestine"—he pointed to the duodenum, pancreas, associated ducts, and the surrounding lymph nodes—"is simply indistinguishable from the surrounding tissue." The mass extended up into roughly 75 percent of my liver—about fifteen tumors of all sizes. The tumors in the left lobe of the liver were the size of golf balls, and those in the right lobe were the size of dimes and nickels.

This explanation took only a minute or two. When he glanced over at Kristin, he stopped speaking, and the look on his face told me why. The memory of the look on Kristin's face still grips me by the throat and overwhelms me every time I think of it.

Her entire manner was that of a completely terrified ten-year-old girl. She was at the edge of her seat, sitting up straight, staring wide-eyed as tears streamed down her face. Her lips curled into a big frown and quivered as she very softly asked Dr. Matlock, "Our boys aren't going to have a dad?" He did not answer. She turned to me, looked deep into my eyes, and squeaked out in the same voice, "We were supposed to grow old together."

I tightly gripped her hand and just kept repeating in a determined voice that everything would be alright. What the hell did I know.

I was stunned, but not yet overwhelmed. An army credo came to mind: "The first report from the battlefield is always wrong." The reality could be better, it could be worse, but the first report was almost always wrong. As far as I was concerned, we needed to focus on getting the rest of the story, not planning my funeral.

Dr. Matlock then said something sympathetic, but self-evident: "I don't think you're going to be able to go on that deployment."

No shit, doc. No shit.

He suggested the Mayo Clinic in Rochester, just ninety minutes away, but the discussion trailed off, because Mayo was not in my insurance network. I told Kristin we could sort things out at home.

We had driven separately to the appointment because Kristin had come directly from work, and I worried about her driving home alone in such a highly emotional state. I had never seen her so visibly shaken.

When I got home, I walked in the door, primed for an explosion of grief and rage, confusion and fear. I was way off. This unassuming and normally soft-spoken woman had been busy on the phone the whole ride home. During her fifteen-minute drive, she had managed to secure a comprehensive set of appointments two days later at the Mayo Clinic: GI, oncology, and surgery—she had them all.

"We ain't waiting on TRICARE," she said with conviction,

referring to our insurance company. Her tone told me she knew I might object. I asked how she had gotten all of this done without a formal diagnosis or medical referral.

"I wouldn't take no for an answer."

My soldier's heart doubled in size. *That* is an army wife, by God. It was also one of the most powerful examples of strength and courage in the face of fear I have ever seen.

✯ ✯ ✯

Strength. Weakness. Bravery. Fear.

I sometimes wonder if we think too seldom of what these words mean. We're taught early on in life that being afraid is something to be ashamed of. This is wrongheaded. Fear is healthy. Fear keeps us alive. When I went through the army's airborne and air assault schools and learned to jump out of planes and slide down ropes hanging from helicopters, I did not want to be sitting next to any trooper who wasn't just a little afraid about what she was going to do.

Bravery, then, is not about avoiding fear or finding ways to ignore it; it's a reflection of what you intend to do with your fear. Facing it means taking in everything about your situation—the good and the bad—and figuring out what you are going to do about it. Anything else is just a variation of surrender.

Strength is about getting something done, even when you have ironclad excuses or reasons for not doing it. Your mom has a hard time seeing how she exemplifies this, but she had shown it to us every day. She can feel her weakness, and that scares the hell out of her, but as sad and as upset as she is about what life has handed her, she never loses sight of what must be done to care for you, for her job, and for our home.

What will you do when those moments arrive in your life?

CHAPTER ONE

July 2010

The entire medical team at the Mayo Clinic was unanimous in their assessment—*there was no path of comfort.* The team proposed a massive and radical surgery called "the Whipple-plus." The Whipple would remove the mush of what was left of my duodenum, the bile and pancreatic ducts, the head of the pancreas, the surrounding lymph nodes, the gallbladder, and *maybe* more, depending on what they found when they cut me open. The "*plus*" would remove 60 percent of my liver but only half of the cancer, with plans to come back for the rest later.

The doctors were incredibly upbeat, but they offered more conditions and caveats than a car commercial.

Forget the cancer. The surgery alone would result in months of severe physical disability, an overnight change in lifestyle (eating, activity, leisure, work, social interaction), and just as much cancer left inside my body as the doctors planned to take out.

The doctors on my Mayo surgical team performed five Whipples per week, but they didn't conceal their inexperience with the Whipple-plus or sugarcoat its risks. With the surgery, I *might* die soon, they said; without the surgery, I *would* die soon.

It wasn't a hard decision for me. If I was going down, I would go down fighting.

When an army is about to go on the offensive, there is nothing more motivating than a rousing set of remarks from the commanding officer. I decided to rally my small army of supporters in the same way. The inspiration for what to write came to me one morning just as I opened my eyes. By 0600, I was feverishly typing out my own adaptation of General George Patton's remarks to the Third US Army on the eve of D-Day, the largest invasion in world history. My rally read, in part:

At ease! (which means, "listen up!")

Now, I want you to remember that no bastard ever won a war by dying for his country. He won it by making the other poor dumb bastard die for his country. Family, friends, all this stuff you've heard about cancer always winning the fight . . . is a lot of horse dung.

. . . You know, by God, I actually pity those poor cancer cells we're going up against. By God, I do . . . We're going to murder those lousy bastards by the bushel.

. . . Thirty years from now when you're sitting around your fireside with my *grandchild on your knee and he or she asks you what I did in the year 2010, you won't have to say, "Well, he sat around and felt sorry for himself in Minnesota."*

. . . Alright now, you sons-of-bitches, you know how I feel. Be strong with me. Fight with me. Oh, and I will be proud to lead you wonderful guys into battle—anytime, anywhere. That is all.

It was not lost on me that Patton had survived a thirty-six-year army career and two world wars only to suffer an inglorious death from injuries sustained in a car accident four months after the end of the war. Now it looked as if I might survive combat and twenty-one years in the army only to succumb to cancer at age thirty-nine.

War speeches may sound great to adults, but they don't play so well with children. When deciding how and what to tell you boys about the cancer, we decided early on that if you were expected to endure the crash landing, you had better be on board for the takeoff.

Bad news does *not* get better with time. Sooner or later, the people you know and love are going to find out. Who do you want them to hear it from—*you* or *someone else*? And if they hear it from someone else, what are the chances your bad news becomes something worse? (As in, "Why would you keep something this important from me?")

Keeping things quiet until we had more information was not an option for us, because the information was floating on Facebook like a stray bullet. Thankfully, Joshua and Noah were only ten years old and had no cell phone or computer, and Matthew, you were in New Mexico at the Philmont Boy Scout camp, where there was no reception. We needed to get to you before the news did—but *not* before you finished your camp.

Philmont is a rite of passage for scouts, and you were only a day or two from completing it as a fourteen-year-old. You had already hiked seventy-five miles and seven mountain peaks (with 8000-to-9000-foot elevation) with a fifty-pound pack over eleven days—every single day in some rain, and three full days in rain and fog. The last thing I wanted you to hear as you reveled in this amazing achievement was an accidental, "Hey, sorry about your dad" from one of your comrades or scout leaders.

My deployment provided a perfect cover story, and I swear I could hear the theme song to *Mission: Impossible* in the background as we went to work. We ensured you were whisked away as soon as you came off the trail, and then we disabled your phone and shut down your Facebook page.

With all you boys home, and with a diagnosis and plan in hand for what would come next, we broke the news. In reflecting upon "what" and "how much" to share, it was helpful to remind ourselves that entire books had been written on this subject. We knew we had to separate the things that needed to be addressed now from the things that could be addressed later.

One question ended up guiding our thinking: *What are you going to see or hear in the next two to four weeks?*

Since there's almost five years of age between you, we told you separately—first Matthew, then all three of you together. We gave you the same message but presented it in different ways, based on your age and personality. Because of our army life, this wasn't the first time we'd had the "what if something really bad happens to Dad" talk. And before each of my deployments, we had discussed the immense responsibility you needed to assume while I was away, *whether I survived or not.*

I organized my thoughts in writing and rehearsed before talking to you. "Boys, I know you're smart little buggers, and you've probably noticed a lot of stuff going on around you this past week, right?"

Noah, you slowly nodded and commented, "I have seen Mom's face looks red around the eyes a lot." You also commented about the number of sad people you saw coming and going. You added, "And I think I heard Grandma Coughlin say something about you and cancer when she was on the phone last week." (I wasn't mad about this misstep, only reminded that kids see and hear more than we think.)

The calm in your voice told me you knew the information but didn't understand it.

"I do have cancer," I said. "I know it doesn't look like it, but I am very, very sick inside."

Your face transformed much like Kristin's had in the doctor's office. You started sobbing and reached for Kristin's leg. I stopped. Joshua and Matthew sat stone-faced, but as introverts, I knew they were processing that same emotion inside. I felt I needed to acknowledge it all before continuing.

"Why are you crying?" I gently asked.

"Because you're gonna *die*," you said as you rolled your eyes.

I tried to address all three of you in my reply. "Well, that's part of why Mom and I are talking with all of you now—to help you understand what's happening. I won't lie to you. I might die soon, but I'm not dead yet, and I have been given a chance that lots of people don't get."

Then I deliberately switched to a stern voice—the one I use for discipline. "I've been given a chance to fight, boys, and that is *exactly* what I'm going to do. You need to know this fight is going to be pretty easy right now—getting smart about this stuff and doing good planning, strategizing, preparing. But it's going to get a *lot* harder. In a few weeks, you're going to see your dad knocked down hard, and I'm going to be in the hospital for a long time. I . . . am going . . . to look . . . *rough*. Those will be the days that I may not look like 'me,' but I'll be in there—*fighting*."

I switched back to a much softer tone. "You may not see me cry much, but I *do* cry. I get scared, and I do get mad about this cancer thing. You're probably going to experience those same feelings, and you need to know that's okay. It's okay to be sad, mad, frustrated, scared, and even to enjoy a little denial every once in a while. But you *cannot* stay there."

When I was a young soldier, I explained, we performed training missions that lasted all day and most of the night for up to a week at a time. "When someone on the team got tired, we stopped and we took a knee to rest. But we *always* got back up, and we never quit . . . *never*. Just like those young soldiers, we can all take a knee too, but if we don't get back up and move out, we're likely going to die or fall to pieces in that place." I told them soldiers aren't always happy about doing it, but we do what must be done.

This had to be done, too. "We're all going to get through this together as a team."

We continued, discussing the healthy things you could do, like talking to your school counselor, or swimming or playing to occupy your mind and your energies. We also discussed the unhealthy things you should avoid when "dealing" with your emotions and how vulnerable those emotions would make you.

I'm sure you remember that I took the opportunity, as I usually did with the subject of emotions, to use my Yoda voice from *Star Wars*: "Anger, fear, aggression—the dark side of the Force, they are. Easily they flow, quick to join you in a fight. Consume you, it will, as it did Obi-Wan's apprentice."

You all smiled dismissively, as if this were not the time to joke. "Stop it now, Dad, that's not real," was the reply you gave me, but I know you all love and relate to *Star Wars*. This was *your* language.

Although a smile would have been nice to lighten the mood a bit, I was dead serious about the reference. "Guys," I said, "I know *Star Wars* isn't real, but it *is* a story written by real people who understand emotions. What they wrote for Yoda about Anakin Skywalker is true, and his warning applies to all of us."

I then shared the story of my younger cousins, Michael and Katie Bryant. You knew Michael was a doctor and that he was helping me navigate the medical hurdles following my diagnosis. I explained that when Michael was seven years old, his dad was killed horrifically and instantly in a head-on collision with a semi-tractor trailer. He didn't get a chance to say or do anything with his dad after that terrible accident.

What did Michael choose to do with his emotion and energy? He became a doctor. And his little sister became a lawyer.

Part of me desperately wanted to shield you from the pain and suffering. I decided against it, because I don't think you or *any* child needs a shield. In fact, I think kids are more adaptable and resilient than most adults.

Pain and suffering are inevitable in this life, and shielding you from it won't help when you're on your own—whether I'm dead or not. What you need more than anything is a shepherd, so that's what Kristin and I offered.

My focus since the diagnosis is no different than it was before the diagnosis—to help you think about how to navigate the hardships you're certain to face in life, not how to avoid them.

☆ ☆ ☆

I doubt my grandparents would say they *wanted* to face the difficulty and challenge of life during the Great Depression and World War II, as MacArthur implies we ought to do. They had little choice about "paths of comfort."

You, however, are likely to face a different world and life circumstances than they did, which means you will have far more choices when it comes to comfort or difficulty (just as I did). What my grandparents taught me through their lack of choice about facing difficulty was that there would be virtue in my choice to face difficulty.

Marie Lanoux married my grandpa, Matt Garofalo, in 1947 when they were both thirty-one years old. Despite a relatively late start, she bore fifteen children over the next fifteen years—with a set of twins for good measure. (The doctor delivered Marco for free, because he made a dozen.)

In 1981, when she was sixty-three and her youngest was just graduating from high school, she suffered a stroke and spent the next seventeen years half-paralyzed and in a wheelchair. I was nine years old at the time, and those years remain an unparalleled example of how to face a *no-choice* hardship with dignity and grace.

Every week, my mom drove the two miles to Grandma's house to visit and help for at least a few hours. I loved coming along to help make Grandma her oatmeal and poached egg or ride my bike to Cossetta's Deli to get sandwiches for lunch.

I was also a chatty kid, so a visit from me always included a fair amount of friendly conversation about nothing in particular. The only time I heard her raise her voice was to plead for one of her adult children to come downstairs and take her to the bathroom. This observation was more than casual for me at age eleven. *What would it be like to have to rely on someone to take me to the bathroom?*

When I was fourteen years old, I started asking if I could help more—and not just with the dishes or meals. I wanted to be able to take care of that bathroom request as soon as she had it. Doing so was no easy task. Grandma weighed at least 160 pounds, and she wasn't able to pull down her own undergarments. I can't think of a more humbling task for a fourteen-year-old boy and his sixty-seven-year-old grandma, but she showed no shame, so neither did I. The task needed to be done.

I helped make meals, did laundry, cleaned dishes, vacuumed, mopped the kitchen floor, and grocery shopped. When I got older and could drive, I visited her during day-trips to the local nursing home. We painted ceramics and played cards, bingo, and cribbage with her friends. She loved showing me off to the other residents, and I enjoyed receiving unbounded appreciation from someone who wanted and needed my small dose of help so badly.

As aware as I thought I was of Grandma's condition at the time, I can look back and see that I was clueless. She took enough medication to choke a horse. Her feet were horribly swollen. And her recliner was a virtual prison when she was alone.

If she ever voiced a complaint, I don't remember hearing it. But I do not consider it noble that she suffered in silence; I consider it noble that she focused her actions and thoughts on *life*, which helped her cope with the suffering.

When I was in my mid-twenties and could better grasp the profound difficulty of her situation, I said to her, "For fifteen years,

I've seen you live your life in that recliner or in your wheelchair. I can tell that you suffer. What the hell keeps you going every day?"

She didn't smile or say a word. She just raised her good arm and pointed to the walls all around her at the more than two hundred photos covering every square inch of space in the small living room: all her children, every wedding, more than thirty grandchildren and some of their wedding photos, and then great-grandchildren as well.

A path of comfort was not an option for her, but she defined what it meant to face the stress and spur of difficulty and challenge.

* * *

If my grandma taught me compassion, endurance, and patience, Grandpa Mathew Garofalo (Mat) must have taught me the value of unbridled passion and the idea that challenge could be fun (albeit in a very odd way).

He was a tall, thin, tireless, remarkably loud, and foul-mouthed automobile mechanic who ran his own repair shop out of his two-car home garage well into his eighties.

He was drafted for World War II, but he saw no honor in the task—then or later. He believed his greatest triumph of the war was that his family convinced the War Department to send him home to Minnesota to take care of his Italian-speaking parents shortly after being drafted. Even in hindsight, he didn't think a world war held as much sway as taking care of his family. And it seemed his harshest words were saved for those who didn't see it the same way (which did not help me when I joined the army).

Despite his deep conviction about family, he had a strange way of expressing affection. "I should have had pigs," he was fond of telling his kids in later years. "At least I could eat them." His temper (our family prefers the word *passion*) was legendary. On two separate occasions, he entered his home in a tirade and smashed his entire dining room set to pieces for reasons known only to him.

Passion, I guess.

Mat's personality was so consistent and predictable that he was virtually a Disney character (PG-13, at best). The only time he made an appearance inside the house was during mealtime. Otherwise he was in the garage or in the basement working. "You don't work, you don't eat," he was fond of saying.

His "office" was the basement, a cavernous, damp dungeon filled wall to wall and floor to ceiling with car parts, tools, brass fittings, and barrels of footwear from the junkyard. A single, winding goat path spanned the fifty-foot length of the room. In a tiny unfinished corner, there was a rudimentary shower stall that looked as if it had been imported from a third world mud hut. He would request things from upstairs by banging on a pipe with a wrench and shouting his demands.

He blacktopped his thirty-by-forty-foot backyard, reasoning it would not require mowing (despite his abundance of free labor). By the time the Weber boys came along, his backyard consisted of nothing but stacks of tires and a massive doghouse for his German wolfhound, Igor.

Mat's "lectures" were always a show, too. No matter what the topic, he included at least one curse word and repeated his explanations at least twice. Since he always talked this way, we just accepted it. I don't remember thinking "angry," as much as I thought "poetry." Any common annoyance could set him off. A normal rant might include something like, "Johnny doesn't listen. Doesn't . . . Fuckin' . . . Listen. Nope. Can't listen. Doesn't know how to listen. Wouldn't know how to listen if his *life* depended on it. If his life depended on listening, he would be dead." All at maximum volume and directed toward no one person in particular. In fact, the offending party was usually long gone by the time he got rolling.

With fifteen kids under the same roof, he took on the disciplinary style of a quirky prison camp captain. He integrated his work and his family life by using a fan belt for whippings. Lining up his young offenders, he would graciously ask, "Do you want a Chevy, Ford, or Pontiac?"

Mat's physical appearance was deceiving. Even in his sixties, he moved like a tall version of Yoda—slightly hunched over and methodical in a routine, but lightning fast in a dustup with one of his teenage boys. He was known to chase one or more of them in the back alley or out into the neighborhood to exercise his judgment.

From my earliest memories I can recall from when my brothers and I visited, he would yell in a deep voice from the garage, "Oh boy, here we go. *Here we gooo!* Open a keg'a nails. *Nail everything down!*" He did this without even pulling his head from under the hood. Again, he didn't sound angry, but he never sounded happy either. We never knew exactly how he felt or quite what he meant, but his ranting always made us smile.

Conversations with Grandpa Garafalo would be about one of two subjects—cars or sex. I'm sure we talked about other things, but I'll be damned if I can remember what. Examples? He spoke of women he'd known before marriage as "conquests," using Italian words for his manhood or for sexual acts. One routine sex reference was known simply as "box of bananas," a throwback to the days when he'd come home for lunch and throw a box of bananas on the kitchen table to keep all the kids busy while he spent some private time with Grandma.

He lived until age ninety-two, when I was stationed in Minnesota. He was the only grandparent I personally watched waste away, and his struggle less than two years before my cancer fight provided a timely example.

When I laid him down on the floor to perform some range of motion exercises with his legs, he casually told me something that illustrated how *he* was going to face the end of his life. With fire and conviction in his voice, he said, "There's only one thing I want to do when I'm in this position."

During his eulogy, the church erupted in gasps and laughter when I pointed out that Saint Peter is likely still wondering who threw a box of bananas up on the lectern while running past him at a sprint.

* * *

Grandma Weber (Marie)—my favorite grandparent as a young boy—had a deep impact on me for completely different reasons than those of my other grandparents. She died at age sixty-seven of a heart attack—on a Sunday morning just before Easter Mass.

Life doesn't get much more ironic or devastating for a twelve-year-old Catholic boy.

We found out much later in life that she suffered from bipolar disorder—really high "highs" and really low "lows." Beyond a few notable examples involving a flying coffee cup (with coffee in it) and some cursing episodes, all I remembered was a sweet, old woman whom I loved more than anyone else in my life.

The day Grandma Weber died was deeply spiritual for me. Her loss made no sense at all. I asked a lot of questions of God. *Why Easter Sunday of all days? Was this a punishment? Were we, or I, not faithful enough?*

I was a frustrated young boy who firmly believed what I was taught—that God could fix anything if I prayed hard enough. Clearly life, as beautiful as it could sometimes be, didn't work that way.

* * *

Grandpa Francis Weber's story is also one of dramatic difficulty and challenge. "Franny" was a cocky and handsome bachelor all through his twenties, and I could tell from our many conversations he thought he lived too fast and loose with alcohol and women (though he never shared any details). At around age thirty, when the idea of family was still a distant thought, he was involved in a bizarre construction accident that nearly killed him.

Franny was a carpenter, but he worked most of the trades, including masonry. The work that nearly ended his life involved tuck pointing damaged brick on a commercial building. Back then, masons used a rudimentary scaffolding system that involved pulleys, boatswain seats, wooden wedges, and planks.

His descriptions and rough drawings of these setups appeared to me like an archeological dig site in an Indiana Jones movie. It was hard to picture such a setup in the mind's eye, but those were spartan times, and this was long before the existence of the Occupational Safety and Health Administration. If we didn't have an actual picture of him standing on such a contraption suspended eight stories in the air, we wouldn't have believed it was possible.

For reasons Franny couldn't explain, his partner and boss that day pulled a support wedge that triggered a collapse of the system beneath their feet. He said his fingertips just brushed the edge of a safety rope as he slid off the plank and plunged eighty-four feet to the ground below into a massive pile of brick, mortar, and wooden planks. He landed on top of his boss, who died at the site.

He broke nearly every bone in his body, including his legs and hips. The impact popped one of his eyeballs out of the socket and left one of his ears dangling from the side of his head. He was so badly injured that the hospital staff didn't know what to do with him.

When he regained consciousness, he was on a gurney in the hallway of the hospital with no one around. He told us he figured no one expected him to survive his wounds, so they just set him aside to die; after all, this *was* a Depression-era hospital in the 1930s.

He spent three months in a full-body cast, and the injuries he sustained would plague him for the rest of his life. His wrist remained disfigured, and his torso looked as if it had been reattached to his body off-center.

When I was an adolescent, this unbelievable story seemed to

be the great catastrophe of Franny's life. As a man, however, I saw something very different: he spent fourteen years suffering from depression after Grandma died, and it got worse as he got older. Though he was physically able until he died at ninety-one, my family had to goad him to take showers, change his clothes, care for his dog, or avoid eating spoiled food.

All through my early twenties, I tried to speak to him about what plagued his mind. "Guilt," he would say. He gave hints of regrets from his youth or his or Grandma's transgressions later in life, but he refused to say more. He just cried.

Now, I don't want to leave you with the picture of a pathetic, sad, old man. Franny remained an incredibly spirited character who had the most unique ways of making us laugh. When he passed gas, he would either say, "Excuse me, I thought I was in Kokomo," or he would call out to an invisible cat, "Here kitty, kitty, kitty." If we ever replied "Huh?" to a question, he replied back with, "Kick a pig in the hind-end, ya get 'huh.'"

Whether inescapable or self-perpetuated, you should know Grandpa Weber's psychological difficulty and challenge plagued him as much or more than his big fall.

✷ ✷ ✷

I suffered pain of my own as a child.

Physically, every kid has issues of one sort or another. Looking back, I see a kid who may have been an example in the extreme: tonsillitis at age two, fourteen years of recurrent ear infections with four corrective surgeries, two broken wrists, dental braces (twice), and eyeglasses at age ten. Each of these troubles is common for children, but I never have seen a kid with all of them.

I was also accident prone, and probably not the right kid to put in the top bunk of beds. Three times I rolled out, breaking my wrist on one occasion and losing a tooth on another. (Oh, there were safety rails back then, but I didn't think I needed those.)

But the ear problems, those were difficult enough to be formative. Every year, I managed to get lake water trapped behind my
eardrum, which caused an infection and immense pressure on the
middle ear. Those tiny bones are so sensitive, I could feel a stinging
pain with each heartbeat, which was ninety thousand beats per day
until the fluids drained and the infection was gone.

Although most kids are given antibiotics or ear drops to clear
up infections, those solutions were not used or didn't work for me.
My doctor didn't like using antibiotics (he thought they were over-
used), and the ear drops were useless. Four times between the age
of five and sixteen, a surgeon cut a small hole in my eardrum and
inserted a small plastic tube, which allowed the fluids to drain.

At least two weeks of every summer were spent writhing in
pain or feverishly pumping my ears with my thumb. Evenings were
a sleepless nightmare. No one complained about my crying, but
I remember moving to different parts of the house so I wouldn't
disturb anyone.

I never did (and still don't) dwell on how these experiences may
have affected me as an adult. As with my grandparents, there was no
choice about a path of comfort, but perhaps I learned more than I
realized about facing the stress and spur of difficulty and challenge.

✳ ✳ ✳

During my freshman year in high school I experienced pain—
at school and at home—that I would have traded for all the ear
infections in the world.

I attended Cretin High School, an all-boys Catholic school.
One of my *least* favorite events was gym class. I loved the activities,
but I hated what came at the end of class—the showers. This was a
particularly stressful event for a Catholic boy whose understanding
of guilt and shame about nudity was as old as Adam and Eve.

The shower ritual felt like a daily walk on thin ice. Since we
were all cut from the same religious cloth, I presumed we each had

an appreciation for the unwritten etiquette: do your business, get out, get dressed, and don't joke about it.

Three months into my freshman year, that etiquette was grotesquely violated, and I was the unlucky and random victim of a cruelty that followed me for the next three years.

Inexplicably, a classmate I didn't even really know raised his head into the air and shouted to the ceiling, "Hey, anybody notice Weber pop a woody in the shower?" He was just six lockers away from me and in my line of sight. I'll never forget the cocky, shit-eating grin on his face after he said it.

I stood there frozen in place, staring wide eyed at my locker. *Do I respond? Do I just stand here? Maybe no one heard him. Just ignore him.*

He repeated his taunt, and it was like being poked with an electric cattle prod. Just then, someone "bit," and other boys joined in the feeding frenzy. I tried making it a joke and said, "Good one, Shane. That's a funny one."

"Whatever, Weber. Don't play it off, man," he replied.

Then he raised his voice to the ceiling again, "Better bring your soap-on-a-rope," he yelled, "and watch out for Webs in the shower . . . he'll sneak up and getcha in the rear." I felt a tingle of shock rush through my chest as I darted out of the locker room and prayed to God that was the end of it.

It was only the beginning.

The comments and ribbing continued for the remainder of that year and my sophomore year, and then lingered through my junior year after we merged with an all-girls school and became Cretin-Derham Hall.

It's hard to describe such an experience without overstating *or* understating it. I wasn't grilled constantly by most kids on most days. It was just a steady drumbeat of ridicule, with the gaps between incidents filled with fear.

Nothing I said or did—laugh about it, remain silent, reply

with "whatever," point out that no one else saw it happen, threaten to fight the offender—made the nightmare go away. When verbal taunts didn't seem to rile me enough, someone etched "Woody" and "Woodman" on my locker.

My mom wanted to get the administration involved, but that brought visions of new taunts such as, "Look who needed his mommy to come fix things for him."

Life would never again present me with a social problem quite as painful or unsolvable. Although I never want to repeat the experience, hindsight reveals a welcome consequence: I was practicing skills in conflict management that served me well for the rest of my life.

Freshman year brought an extraordinary amount of stress at home as well. Mom had had enough of Dad's drinking and the effect it was having on our family. He wasn't a mean drunk or a hard drinker, but his drinking was more than a distraction. It was affecting his work, another woman was involved, and there was at least one awkward incident in our driveway that almost brought the police. Mom kicked him out of the house and said the only way he was ever coming back was if he stopped drinking.

Four months into an ugly separation, we wondered if he would ever be coming back, and I can honestly say I didn't much care. Though we knew the separation had to do with more than just Dad or the alcohol, it didn't matter. Routinely seeing Mom quietly crying in a dark corner made us angry and fiercely protective.

With all of the problems at home and at school, suicide crept into my head as a possible solution. It was the "easy button," and the very thought of it brought me comfort.

I played out the scenarios in my head in the weeks that followed, and I came to a solid conclusion that suicide actually wouldn't solve a damn thing. I didn't suffer from a mental illness. I was fully capable of facing my difficulties; I just didn't want to anymore.

Given my conditions, I concluded that suicide would be a

selfish and lazy thing to do, and it would only bring more pain to
those I loved. I decided to stick it out.

✯ ✯ ✯

My life as a soldier began when I was a freshman at Cretin
High, which had a military institute tradition dating back a
hundred years.

My early start with army life makes it seem as if this is what I
was born to do. It's difficult to argue against it, but nothing could
be further from the truth. *Every* decision along this twenty-three-
year-long path was a conscious choice that involved a lot of self-
doubt and anxiety.

Nothing about my life story will tell you this, but I was very
apprehensive about army life during those first eight years. And
I was far from a model of discipline and conviction when I first
donned the uniform.

At Cretin, I wasn't some kid embarking on an army career.
I was merely doing what most of the kids from Saint Francis de
Sales Grade School did. The "military program," also known as the
Junior Reserve Officer Training Corps (JROTC), was voluntary,
and I was more than a little anxious about joining. My only frame
of reference was the 1981 movie *Taps*, where the kids took over the
high school and started a small war in their town.

Thankfully, ours was more like a course in leadership and
management. Instructors emphasized citizenship and leadership
development. We explored real-world examples of leadership traits
such as courage, loyalty, dedication, integrity, initiative, and determination. For many friends and family, there was concern that
JROTC would brainwash me into wanting to join the army. They
were *partly* right. I *was* soon brainwashed, but only with "poisoned"
ideas such as:

- Set the example.

- Seek responsibility and take responsibility for your actions.

- Look out for the welfare of the people under your care.

- Know yourself and seek self-improvement.

- Develop a sense of responsibility in your subordinates.

- Officers serve and protect the Constitution, not individual leaders.

- Don't ask your subordinates to do something you wouldn't do yourself.

These were ideals I saw and learned at home and at church, but other ideals—"speak up" or "disagreement doesn't equal disrespect"—were altogether new and not exactly welcome with my parents or the church leadership. So this instruction empowered a young upstart like me. It told me I was not only entitled to seek responsibility and speak out, but that it was noble and honorable to learn how to do it respectfully and with competence.

The meritocracy and hierarchy of the military program brought with it a welcome predictability. We wore the army dress uniform every day, and we were given cadet rank and positions of responsibility.

Our "work" had limited value in the real world—marching and keeping clean and pressed uniforms, neatly trimmed hair, shined shoes, and properly placed awards and decorations—but they *were* very practical ways to demonstrate and evaluate personal responsibility, discipline, and integrity.

Unfortunately, JROTC aroused certain fears among parents and non-JROTC staff. The sight of a mass of kids marching in uniform and dutifully saluting and carrying out "orders" can send a chill up the spine of even the most reasonable adult, and I heard references to Nazi Germany and the Hitler Youth.

Our instructors took note. They were all retired army soldiers and veterans of the wars in Vietnam and Korea. Most of them had been wounded in combat. They personally saw the horrors of war and were quick to humble any student who expressed romantic thoughts about the life of a soldier.

I gave all my attention and energy to the JROTC program, and it showed in good ways and bad. I could march a unit like one of Napoleon's best, recite on demand the meaning of leadership traits and principles, and perform drill with a rifle better than any student in recent memory. But I was an unfocused academic student with an undisciplined mouth.

When I was a junior, I told a teacher to shut up when she said something insulting to me. Today I would call that "good initiative, bad judgment." She was wrong, but telling her to shut up was a too-easy solution with harsh consequences. When the promotion order for lieutenant was published for our class—an important milestone in the program—my name was not listed. I openly wept in front of my friends. It took a few weeks for me to realize the failure was all mine.

As my time at Cretin came to a close, it dawned on me that my four years had produced some spectacular achievements—of little or no practical value. I earned a 2.25 GPA and a 19 on my ACT. I played no sports, performed no volunteer work, and held no major leadership positions in JROTC.

My talents included exceptional debate skills, a solid grasp of leadership and management traits, and the ability to recite the eighty-seven counties of Minnesota from memory in under thirty seconds (don't ask).

My high school counselor was fairly blunt: "College is not for you. I don't even think any college will take you. You should start thinking about what you want to do for a living." That high school counselor's words were a wakeup call: *I need to start thinking more and working harder.*

* * *

When the time came to meet with an army recruiter, the choice seemed as natural as picking out something for dinner. And it wasn't all "duty, honor, and country."

Joining the Minnesota Army National Guard paid for half of my tuition, provided several hundred dollars of income per month, and would help establish a career if I decided to stick with it after graduation from college. Even my choice of army profession (military police) was based on finances—a $2,000 bonus.

Moving from Minnesota to Alabama for basic training was as shocking as being thrown into ice-cold water. Our open sleeping bays were a close-quarters stewpot of personalities, cultures, and social backgrounds from all over the country and a total loss of comfort and familiarity. I knew how to march, shoot, map-read, and recite leadership principles better than most of my drill sergeants, but this wasn't high school, and these were *not* underclassmen.

The pace and style of the drill sergeants made my dad's roughness seem quaint. All my hair was cut off, all my freedoms stripped, and every decision made for me. We weren't even allowed to pee without permission.

Eating took place as a necessary provision of life, period. No socializing.

Failure to follow instructions resulted in a tongue-lashing. And the daily rituals often consisted of at least one "Kobayashi Maru" ("no-win" scenario), where the *intent* was to be unfair.

I later learned there was a purpose to the entire approach: *nothing* goes according to plan in combat. Chaos reigns supreme. If a person can't survive the scripted unfairness and "silliness" of life in a training environment, there is no reason to believe he is capable of doing so anywhere else. But knowing it was scripted never made things much easier.

I was a virtual expert in basic military etiquette, but I knew very little about how to actually function under stress. Our very first lesson was learning to stand at attention, which was child's play for me. But stress turned the task into quantum physics. My heart raced, and I inadvertently tightened my hands into a fist instead of keeping them loose and slightly curled as I'd mastered *years* earlier. One of the instructors caught sight and bit hard. "Hey, lookie this one, drill sergeant!" he screamed to his partners in a deep Southern drawl. "He look like he gonna knock someone out! Unclench doz fists, private, and get inta da proppa position of attention!"

My seventeen weeks of basic training and MP school were filled with noteworthy experiences, but in sum, it is best described as an immersion in life without convenience, comfort, or familiarity.

The entire experience redefined my understanding of adversity and hardship.

At home, going to Sunday Mass had always felt like a chore; in the army, it was an oasis. At home, I could just walk away from or ignore the people who bothered me; in the army, I had to learn how to work with them (and I saw that I could). At home, I didn't think I could function if I didn't get eight hours of sleep; in the army, I realized my body and mind were capable of far more output on half the sleep. In essence, I found perspective, and experiencing it in such a full-throttled way helped me strive to seek it out later in life—whether I was in combat in Iraq or in combat with my own body.

Ultimately, I learned how true and valuable it is to actually live one day at a time. It was the mantra I recited to myself over and over when I was alone with my thoughts in the shower after a grueling session of physical training, in my bunk after a difficult day, or lying under the stars during field training exercises. It worked then. It still works now.

☆ ☆ ☆

Eighteen months before my cancer diagnosis, Kristin watched helplessly as her father battled his prostate cancer during our brief assignment in Minnesota. The cancer had been in remission for years, but it was back, and it seemed to have the upper hand. Faced with uncertainty and an immense feeling of compassion for Kristin, I decided to make a career choice that would cause any career army officer to shudder.

After sixteen years, I resigned my active duty army commission and joined the full-time Minnesota National Guard so our family could remain near him. For once, I wanted Kristin to come before career, when she needed it most.

To say the decision didn't sting would be dishonest. Peers and mentors reacted as if I had committed suicide, and part of me felt as if I had.

I had enjoyed what many considered to be an improbable string of wild successes: national recognition as one of the best junior officers in the army; early promotion to the rank of major, despite an unorthodox career path; selection to attend a fully funded master's degree program at Georgetown University; assignment to the personal staff of the chairman of the Joint Chiefs of Staff; being handpicked by General Petraeus to serve on his personal staff in Iraq; and finally, selection to work in the Office of the Provost Marshal General of the army.

I knew Minnesota would not challenge me professionally in the same way. Worse, there was a blunt reality to joining such a tiny slice of the army. My unique experiences in places like the Pentagon were of little use in Minnesota. And unlike the regular army, where there were over 8,500 lieutenant colonels, Minnesota had only seventeen such positions—*and I would be "the new guy."* I was candidly told that any promotion would be dramatically delayed, if it happened at all.

My decision in light of all this was so unconventional and uncharacteristic that even Kristin was in disbelief until she saw my discharge papers.

I did feel uncertainty and fear about such a dramatic personal and professional shift, but just one look into Kristin's eyes brought comfort in knowing it was the right thing to do.

And the truth is, looking into Kristin's eyes is all the comfort I've ever needed.

✷ ✷ ✷

"I could never do what you have done."

Boys, I've heard this comment countless times during my time in the army, and even more so during my fight with cancer. I'm always hesitant to challenge such well-intentioned comments, but I can tell you a reply does echo inside my head: "Actually, you can do it; you just don't want to do it."

Everyone has things they don't want to do—there's no crime in that. But there's a big difference between "can't" and "don't want to" when it comes to facing the path of comfort or the stress and spur of difficulty and challenge.

I've learned "can't do" is much easier but requires nothing and produces nothing. "Can do," however, will often require you to challenge what you thought you knew, to work with others when you don't want to, to look for perspective where you don't want to look, to risk being wrong, and to actually experience defeat and humiliation. Each of these brings with it the price of learning and living a full and examined life.

I'm not telling you to run out into the oncoming traffic of every difficulty and challenge you set eyes on. I'm proposing that "can do" is often just one or two short steps beyond "can't do," and the territory in between is fertile ground for personal growth and professional achievement.

How sensitive will your "can't" and "don't want to" thresholds be?

CHAPTER TWO

. . . NOT TO SUBSTITUTE WORDS FOR ACTIONS.

August 2010

I open my eyes, and I cannot move. I feel like a piece of dead wood. My head is thick and my vision is foggy. The room is dark with a faint haze of light, just enough so I can make out the various things around me.

I am on my back in a small room with white walls. A large monitor is up to my right, and a shiny, metallic-looking material is along the ceiling in front of me. I slowly turn my head to the left and can make out a US flag. The noises in the room are as faint as the light.

"Where am I?"

I doze off.

When I open my eyes again, I still don't know where I am. A rhythmic swooshing sound is followed by a barely audible, repeating beep. The room is otherwise so silent that I can make out the distinct hum of electronic gear all around my head, as if I'm in a cockpit.

"Dammit, where the hell am I?" The disorientation reminds me

of waking up during a sleepover at a friend's house. But back then, I could figure out where I was. Why can't I figure it out now?

I doze off again.

When I open my eyes again, I am immediately aware of a tapping and clicking noise, and it's happening at a furious rate. I turn my head to the right, and a woman is standing at a console. The light from her monitor gives the room a faint glow. She appears glued to the screen and her task. I ask, "Where am I?" She does not reply. Didn't she hear me? I ask again. No response.

I don't know how much time has passed since I first opened my eyes, but it feels like an hour. Then it hits me. My powers of deductive reasoning have finally kicked in . . . the monitors, the shimmering Mylar, the American flag, all the electronics and the cockpit feeling.

I'm in a spaceship!

I close my eyes, confident in my conclusion. But after just a few moments, I feel disgusted with such thinking. What the hell would I be doing in a spaceship?

I feel a hand on my arm. "How are you doing, Mark?" It is the woman I had seen earlier at the monitor. She looks familiar to me, but I don't know who she is.

"Where am I?" I ask in exasperation. "Why are we in a spaceship?"

She's neither amused nor upset by my question. "You're in the hospital."

My senses are still very dull, but not because it is the middle of the night and I am tired. It's because I am stoned on pain medication. But I finally understand: the woman is my nurse. My eyes well up with tears as I remember this is a nightmare from which I cannot wake up.

I have stage IV cancer, and things have gone from bad to worse as the complications mount from my surgery.

As I lie there completely inactive and having just awakened, my heart beats one hundred times per minute, which is a jogging pace for me. I actually feel as if I've been jogging. It's been banging away nonstop like this since the surgery three weeks ago (and will continue for another four weeks).

I'm aware my internal organs no longer resemble the human design. It's a marvel anything works, but it does. My surgeon explains he's hit some snags in the plumbing redesign. The undamaged part of my pancreas was still healthy—unexpected for pancreatic cancer.

*Sewing a healthy pancreas back onto the intestine is like sewing a banana to a condom. And sewing the Pixy-Stix-size bile duct into place is an equally challenging task. I was warned that approximately 20 percent of Whipples develop a fistula (*intestinal leak*) as a result, and I am a lucky winner.*

In the days following my surgery, I could look down at my abdomen and see a neatly sewn pattern traced along the bottom of my entire rib cage. But not today. The fistula has allowed most of my abdominal cavity, from my ribs to my hip, to fill with bile and pancreatic fluids. Last week, the surgeon had to open all the stitches along the seventeen-inch-wide incision.

Now I look like a cut-open deer carcass.

"Are you going to put the stitches back in?" I ask. "No," the surgeon says. "It may be hard to grasp this idea, but your entire wound has to heal from the inside out—no stitches. It's what we call an open wound."

Telling me this might be hard to grasp is an understatement. One section of the incision is big enough to allow two fists inside my abdomen. The muscle looks like ground hamburger, and it is bathed in a constant yellow ooze of digestive fluids that will require bandage changes every few hours or so (for the next fourteen weeks).

*As I reach down to lift the bed sheet away from my abdomen, I can feel the tug of the tubes hooked to my right arm. I glance up at the four bags of fluid hanging from the IV stand. I cannot eat because my new plumbing can't handle the pressure or the task of processing food. So two of the IV bags provide my only nutrition (*TPN*).*

*A fifth tube runs to a pump of Dilaudid (*morphine times ten*), which I can control. It comes with a detonator-like button I hit with my* *thumb when the pain becomes too much, which is about once an hour.*

One of the side effects of the pain medication is the worst cotton mouth I've ever experienced in my life. But even worse than that is the fact that I can't drink anything, and I feel thirsty twenty-four hours per day. The only water I'm allowed is ice chips or a moist sponge to keep my lips from drying out. (I wasn't allowed to drink until day twenty.)

I think about how long it takes for a small cut on my hand to heal, and then I look down at that big incision. "There's no freakin' way, man," I whisper.

The weeks that preceded and followed this single day were pure torture—one problem snowballing into another. The heavy narcotics, massive abdominal wound, drains, and lack of nutrition made it difficult to get out of bed, let alone walk, pee, or pass gas.

Every day, I would stand and plead with God for that pee to flow, because a nurse with a catheter was the only alternative if it didn't. You can imagine how painful it might be to have a catheter pushed up the urethra of my penis three times a day to drain the bladder.

"Can't you just leave the damned thing in there instead of cramming it in and out every day?" I begged the nurse.

"Not if you ever want to be able to pee again."

To keep my digestive system moving, prevent blood clots, and maintain *any* kind of muscle in my body, I was required to walk. I couldn't physically do it as often as I needed to, but I tried my best. I shuffled in slow motion for a couple hundred feet or so—one painful step at a time.

My inactivity and "sleepy" organs made it harder for fluids to drain, which resulted in about thirty-five pounds of water-weight gain. My legs and feet were swollen beyond recognition, and my testicles swelled to the size of an orange. (Noah laughingly referred to my genitals as "Big Daddy" after he accidentally caught a glimpse when I climbed into bed.)

The fluid retention also restricted my breathing, which led to fluid buildup on my lungs, all of which made it even harder to walk, sleep, or even think straight. I felt like a bloated deer tick. "Can't you just drain the fluid off the lungs?" I asked.

No. The procedure was too risky. "It would be better if you worked harder with those deep-breathing exercises ten times per day," I was told.

I laughed. I could barely perform them twice per day. Doctors eventually drained a two-liter bottle of fluid out of my lungs.

⋆ ⋆ ⋆

When you're scared, you go with what you know. As a twenty-two-year career soldier and officer, I initially recoiled at the idea of using words like *battle*, *war*, or any other military term to describe the cancer experience. There's a "war" on everything these days—drugs, Christmas, obesity, illiteracy, poverty, terror—and we never seem to win.

I also didn't like the idea that a war reference implied an enemy and losers. Cancer wasn't some foreign invader. It was the result of my own faulty immune system, and I sure wasn't going to consider *myself* the enemy or a loser because of it. Plus, I had seen too many soldiers fight and lose *real* battles in combat with a *real* enemy. It just didn't seem right to make the comparison.

My resistance to using combat-related terms was short lived. Nearly everyone who spoke to me used the metaphor, and the reasons made sense as I gained more perspective from my own disease.

Cancer isn't something that pops, breaks, wears out, or busts loose in your body. It *is* a war—a murderous *civil war* within the body. I found that families with cancer *needed* the metaphor, because terminal diseases like mine tap into our worst nightmares about life—the idea of a slow death and eventually a painful, miserable existence for survivors *and* their caregivers.

The metaphor provided a rallying point for families desperately trying to cope. And as a soldier, war-fighting language was *my* language.

I was once asked to describe the difference between fighting cancer and fighting in combat. (Well, bullets and bombs, for starters.) The only real difference with cancer is the scenery and the fighters, because with cancer, you still have to face an enemy and your own fears. You still have to face death. You still have to endure misery and deprivation, both trivial and severe. And you still have to sit down with family and explain the blunt reality of the possibilities.

So, if everyone characterizes cancer as civil war, and you heard that one million of your own fellow citizens (cancer cells) were moving across the country, indiscriminately killing everyone in their path, whom would you categorize as your "friendly forces" in the fight?

Answer: *Everyone who's not with them.*

In army-speak, my friendly forces consist of three "branches"— my body, my friends and family, and my doctors.

The only *physical* fighter in that lineup is my body. Other people can help, but the actual fighting has to be done by the body and the mind. In July 2010, the massing enemy force wasn't at my border; the cancer already had me outflanked, outgunned, and surrounded. The engine and fuel-processing station (the digestive tract) for my entire fighting force was already destroyed. My body possessed a strong heart, mind, lungs, and muscles, but without fuel, these were just accessories. They were being robbed of their combat capability by the day.

The "friends and family" branch of my army grew by about one thousand "enlistments" in just one week via my online journal.[1] These troops were long in motivation and spiritual support,

---

1.   www.caringbridge.org. Site name: "markmweber." This is a free-access website where all visitors, even those already with an account, must register as a security precaution against those who would seek to prey on our family's circumstances.

but they could not offer any practical fighting capability against the cancer.

The last remaining branch of my army, and the one that possessed the most reason for optimism, was a small team of special forces (my medical doctors) armed with the deadliest, most advanced weapons known to human biology. The problem:

- doctors' weapons kill just as indiscriminately as the cancer;

- the confusion and uncertainty of "the fog of war" is just as unforgiving to doctors;

- doctors' solutions are sometimes entirely ineffective, despite a breathtaking swath of destruction to the cancer.

Any questions?

✳ ✳ ✳

Folks who wanted to support me clearly struggled with what to say outside of "you can beat this—fight like hell!" and "I'll pray for you." It forced me to ask myself some questions about what kind of support I wanted: *I am taking this on like a soldier, but does that mean I want to be told I will be victorious, no matter what? I laugh a lot, but is there anything to laugh about here? I am a spiritual person, but will my faith dictate my survival?*

I decided to tell people my thoughts about each of these subjects and suggest how they could help with each—a task I now consider a responsibility of those who are severely ill. Here's what I told them:

Help me "keep it real" by talking with me about what I can plainly see with my own two eyes. Don't put me in the grave, but don't make boastful claims about my impending victory, either. *Just talk or sit with me.*

With regard to humor, I laugh at myself and at life. This is what

I was like before the cancer, and I have no plans to change now.

When it comes to spirituality (by far the largest offer of support), please respect my beliefs enough not to impose yours. God is my inspiration for fighting and living, but I don't see him as a cosmic bellhop who's going to come loosen my bowels when I can't poop or convince my immune system to start recognizing cancer cells. Pray with me, but please don't tell me you prayed for God to do any work *for* me (or for the doctors). I'm satisfied with the raw materials he gave us at conception and the inspiration he has provided since. *That* is miraculous enough.

☆ ☆ ☆

There came a time when bold talk surrendered to sober reality about the journey and the work that lay ahead. Some thoughts I shared with very few people. *Stage IV cancer is stage IV cancer.* There's no sugarcoating that, no matter how confident and positive a person can be on the outside.

Modern medicine gave me plenty of hope, but I also knew I needed to be honest with myself about the undeniable mortality of my situation. I knew too many people who gained little or nothing in their big fights, spent the next six to eighteen months losing their dignity and most of their quality of life from surgical complications, and then died a slow and painful death.

Some friends and family considered this unhealthy thinking. But to me, this is what "strong enough to know you are weak" and "facing the stress and spur of challenge" really mean. I felt I needed to think long and hard about how I was going to balance my actions with my words.

My reflections and observations didn't sap my courage; they just forced me to consider the possibilities and stay focused on what I needed to *do* (versus what I might dare to "hope for"). The fear of such outcomes motivated me to get smart on the complications following my surgery, to brace myself mentally for things to get

worse, to learn what questions to ask, to review and fully acknowledge my own responsibilities in the effort, and to help my family
seek out the same perspective.

Examples of these considerations in action? I insisted on
packing the open cavity in my abdomen with gauze and changed
all of my own bandages. I demanded to know what medicines were
being pumped into me every day. I read and I learned as much as
I could so I could make independent judgments about all of it—
thicker, thinner, more, less, or not at all.

In order to personalize the fight, I gave names to my wounds
that I still use today. Buford was the open wound. Bullah was the
drainage field inside my abdomen and associated incision at my
hip. (Buford is now the name I use collectively to describe the
entire hardship.)

When I could finally start eating and my "hot" food arrived
cold day after day, I didn't just complain; I asked to see the hospital's kitchen manager and passionately pleaded for better service for
all of us "prisoners." (And he delivered.)

When members of my surgical team talked down to me or
dismissed my explanations of what I was experiencing, I firmly
reminded them I was *part* of the team.

Action didn't always come easy, and that's what teammates are
for. On August 27, Kristin showed up with a towel and some soap
and encouraged me to tackle my greatest fear—the shower. My
first in twenty-five days. I dreaded the *idea* of the pain that could
come from rushing water through my open wounds.

I could barely lift my arms, so I just stood there while Kristin
gently washed every inch of me with a small cloth. "Okay, lift your
leg for me now." I'd imagined a moment like this might come for
one of us during our lives, but not *now*.

She patted me dry when we were done, peeled sheets of dead
skin from my legs and ankles (the result of the swelling), rubbed
lotion on my legs and feet, and dressed me in a clean gown. Then

she crawled into my small bed for the first time since the surgery, and we cuddled. I never felt so secure and comforted in all my life.

It was our sixteenth wedding anniversary.

☆ ☆ ☆

In basic training, my drill sergeant asked me if I thought I could make it through a rigorous obstacle course. "I hope so," I said.

"I'll tell you what, private," he sneered. "You go ahead and hope in one hand and shit in the other, and then tell me which one fills up first."

Since I've commanded my own audiences, I've used a more polite way of demonstrating the power that actions can have over words. I ask them to make an "OK" sign with their forefinger and thumb and then tell them to place the circle on their chin. Ninety percent of the participants instead place the OK sign on their *cheek*. Why? Because I place my own OK sign on *my cheek* while I explain the instruction.

People see what I do and ignore what I say. As people usually do.

Like all lives, mine is *filled* with examples of the power of actions over words—lessons that don't come from instruction manuals.

When I was in JROTC some twenty-eight years ago, a high-ranking senior classman with long hair and a messy uniform didn't wield much influence with lesser-ranked cadets, no matter how competent and motivated he was.

In basic training, we had a bright and confident West Point lieutenant who faced the same dilemma. He could talk articulately and with passion about fitness, soldiering, and leadership. Yet his words were overshadowed by his obesity, and he never seemed to realize it.

It wasn't just hypocrisy that spoke volumes. I noted many drill sergeants ate before their soldiers at mealtime. Considering their workload, no one would have faulted them for doing so. But Drill Sergeant Paradeis ate last. "When I'm done, you're done," he would yell daily. *How could I complain about how little time I had to eat when this guy had less time than me?* When we did physical training, he did it with us (as opposed to standing over us, barking orders). When we went for a six-mile road march, he went the full distance (as opposed to meeting us at the finish line). His simple acts just made me *want* to follow him.

The influence of those decades-old memories informed my behavior throughout my life: *I eat last, and I don't ask anyone to do something I wouldn't do myself.*

✷ ✷ ✷

Nothing underscores the raw simplicity of actions and words like parents and parenting (or any interaction between adults and children). There's not much sense arguing with a ten-year-old who calls you out when your actions don't match your words. *You've kept me humble in this regard, boys, and your kids will do the same, if you let them.*

I judged my parents' actions, too. My mom was *all* nurturer, and her actions as parent were the complete opposite from Dad. She prided herself on being physically *there* for us all the time and showered us with physical expressions of affection. But when it came to consequences, she mostly just threatened. She would call out for my dad when she lost her patience, but then immediately regret the fury she had unleashed.

What my mom lacked in authority because of her familiarity, she gained in trust and confidence. We had mother-son talks—lots of them. Conversations with her were the closest thing I had to a "Dear Diary." I felt free to share my emotions, even if I knew they were irrational. I was a "mama's boy," which I was less embarrassed about once I learned Generals Patton, MacArthur, and Eisenhower all shared the same descriptor.

Love—*an emotion expressed with or for people you always want to be around*—came easy with Mom.

* * *

Love was not a word I would ever have associated with my dad when I was young.

How my brothers and I didn't end up murdered is beyond me. All indications are that we deserved it. I once heard my dad yell that we owed him at least $15,000 for all the doors, vehicle interiors, tools, and home furnishings we damaged or destroyed.

When I was eight or nine, something snapped inside my dad that showed us he was all done with words. I don't remember what triggered it, but I sure remember what happened. In our Minnesota home, there was no shortage of hockey sticks.

He grabbed one, cut off an eighteen-inch section, sat down at the kitchen table, and carved it into the instrument we knew forever after as "the Stick." He even engraved our names on it— *Mike, Mark, Chris*—for added effect.

I don't remember how many times we "got the Stick," but if it happened five times, it happened fifty. Just the *idea* of the Stick was breathtaking. We once tried to hide it, but that didn't work worth a damn.

As a carpenter, it's unlikely my dad was ever introduced to the academic concept known as the "prisoner's dilemma," but he was a natural: "The first one to find the Stick *won't* get a swat with it," or "Tell me who hid it, or you're all going to get it," he'd say.

Threatening to cry child abuse was fruitless. "Pack your bags. If you think this is abuse, I'll drive you to the foster home myself," he said, with Mom's approval. We only played that card once, because we knew he never hit us hard enough to even leave a mark.

"I love you" was neither something my dad said nor something I would have believed if he had said it. He spent most of his time in the garage working on his race car, fishing or hunting, or playing softball. He wasn't an absent father; he was just always busy with other things. We were welcome to tag along if we wanted, but there were no fond entreaties from him.

And if we went along, we'd better bring lunch and a roll of toilet paper, because it was going to be a marathon.

When I was about twelve, I went ice fishing with him. I started feeling ill. I knew better, but I asked if we could go home. "You can wait in the truck, if you want," he said, "but we're not going anywhere." (He told me years later the fish must have been biting.)

As I sat in our truck in that mid-January Minnesota cold, my colon started to rumble. I leapt from the truck and peeled off my coveralls as quickly as I could. *Too late.* The lumpy diarrhea bounced off my leg and flowed straight into my pants. No toilet paper and no spare clothes. My choices were to sit in the poo or strip off my clothes and sit in the truck half-naked. The cold left me no real choice. There was little sympathy when Dad finally returned to the truck.

I suppose I should have learned my lesson from that incident, but several years later, I went with him on an ice fishing trip to Lake Mille Lacs during a fairly warm winter. We drove out onto the ice. The weather was beautiful. We were so far out on the lake, we could barely make out the shoreline. Imagine my horror as I watched our family car sink into the ice up to the middle of the wheels. He calmly explained why we had nothing to worry about, and we did drive off the lake, but that was the last time I went ice fishing with Dad.

Deer hunting was no picnic, either. While early November is not technically winter in Minnesota, it can stand in until winter arrives. At age fourteen, Dad put me in the same clothes he wore when he was young: a couple shirts and a jacket, long underwear and jeans, wool socks, and a pair of tennis shoes with rubber galoshes stretched over them. (Hey, it had been good enough for him at that age.) And *that* was the last time I went deer hunting until I could purchase my own cold-weather gear.

As much as these things bothered me, I couldn't help but be inspired. Nothing seemed to faze my dad—physically or emotionally. His single-minded sense of purpose was something I came to greatly admire as an adult. But as a teenager, the virtue was lost on me, so I nicknamed him "Psycho Daniel Boone," a title he still wears *proudly*.

I don't recall any philosophical "father-son talks." My sense was that he instinctively kept a distance to prevent appearing soft or getting too familiar.

Nurturing and loving were Mom's jobs.

☆ ☆ ☆

There's certainly something to be said about the differences between men and women, or boys and girls, in all of this reflection about choices with words, actions, and parenting. Kristin had no brothers, and she would frequently admit to being at a complete loss about how to judge the behavior of you boys.

It would be irresponsible to leave the descriptions above as examples of what I think are good or bad qualities in a parent. As you can see, there are tradeoffs with parenting styles, as I learned when I practiced them with you.

As rough as my dad was, the soldier in me saw virtue in his approach. Familiarity *does* breed contempt, so instilling a healthy sense of fear and distance counted for a lot when dealing with an immature, undisciplined, or ill-reasoned mind.

But did he—or I—need to abandon affection and playfulness altogether?

On the one-year anniversary of my cancer diagnosis, we tested this question together while we played a board game. But not just any board game. This was Risk, a game that carried some personal history for us.

When you were much younger and we played the same game, I would don some sort of military headgear and use different accents of the region or country being attacked or invaded. You would always look at me like stunned fish—half-confused, half-amused, and always a little embarrassed for some reason. Obviously you were curious, but you never begged me to do the voices, and I never really could tell if you liked it.

Part of the reason for my play-acting was to show you, with my actions, that you're never too old to let your guard down, be playful, and laugh—and that I wasn't hesitant about sharing *some* familiarity with you.

For *this* year's game, I explained that each of *you* was going to dress up with your own headgear. The initial response was skepticism. If I wanted to act like a fool, fine, but that didn't mean you had to do it. Matthew, you broke the ice with some suggestions, and your informal leadership quickly brought Joshua and Noah in tow. Within minutes, you were arguing over the available characters.

I made you all generals and gave each of you a name. Never one to miss a teaching opportunity, I made sure to share a little culture and background about the meaning of the names.

Josh was a Kurdish Peshmerga general named Mustafa Zibari. Peshmerga is the name given to Kurdish fighters (literal meaning, "those who face death"). Zibari is the family name of General Babakir Zibari, the Iraqi officer I worked for in Iraq. Mustafa is the name of the "Kurdish George Washington" of the 1930s and '40s, a man who was largely responsible for maintaining a Kurdish identity within the mostly Arab Iraq.

Matthew was an African general named Kujo Khat. Kujo is the name of a gospel singer in Africa (Matthew sings and plays the guitar). Khat is the name of a flowering plant in the Horn of Africa people of the region chew like tobacco (but with a far more potent effect).

Noah was a Saudi general named Prince Ali Sultan bin Mohammed al Quadari, a name that provided an illustration of Arab culture. Prince Sultan was the name of the crown prince of Saudi Arabia when I was deployed there in 1996. Arabs traditionally do not have first, middle, or last names, but instead carry a string of names with "bin" meaning "son" and "al" meaning "the." So, Noah's name meant, "Ali Sultan, son of Mohammed the Quadari." (An Arab scholar might quibble, but I know I was close enough for this game!)

Finally, I made myself an Australian general, the accent and larrikin attitude of choice for me.

Our three-hour Saturday epic went by fast, until, as with real war, someone had to suffer the humiliation of defeat. The heartache surrounding Prince Ali's demise was pronounced—Noah, you wanted to quit.

I put on my best Aussie accent and offered a lesson with a little humor and grace: losing didn't need to be shameful, but quitting would be, and it wasn't going to happen as long as I was at the table.

"Ya gonna have to play through, mate, that's the only option!" This all resulted in cackles from Matthew and Joshua, but only scornful looks from you, Noah. I recognize this may seem like cruel teasing, but the lesson was sound. And it is a testament of sorts that many months later, all of you recalled the details of the interaction with clarity and pleasure.

Playing Risk made me realize how I am both like and unlike my own father:

Risk, like my dad: The my-way-or-the-highway nature of the enterprise, the demand that Noah finish the game, the not knowing—and ultimately, not caring—if you enjoyed the game.

Risk, unlike my dad: The decision to take the time to do it all in the first place, the playful theatrics, the humor, the cultural curiosity, and the willingness (if impatience) to help an immature mind process emotions in a mature way.

✳ ✳ ✳

A different father-son experience provides a more intense illustration of the question regarding familiarity.

When we returned to Minnesota and experienced our first real winter, my mind wandered back to my childhood. I remembered seeing huge, carved-out snow forts big enough to walk into—projects that required a dad's help. I didn't regret that my dad didn't do this with us, but I wanted to do it with you.

Snowfall is tricky. You can get thirty inches a year, but if the weather isn't cold enough, or it all doesn't fall at the same time, it's difficult to build a snow fort of any decent size.

In December 2009, we hit the jackpot—the fifth largest snowstorm on record in Minnesota, with seventeen inches of snow in one day. Within a week, we got another sixteen inches on top of that. And the timing was perfect—Christmas school break.

I gathered you together as if we were planning the D-Day invasion. "Boys, this is it. This kind of snow comes along once in a kid's lifetime." In fact, a search of Minnesota records revealed only two times in my life when this much snow fell in one day or one month, and one of those times was in December 1982, when I was just one year older than both of you, Joshua and Noah.

Your eyes burned with excitement at the time. But I was not naïve. I knew keeping you motivated would not be easy as the work got harder.

It took me two days to gather the snow from our driveway *and* our neighbor's. At one point, the snow became too packed to move by snowblower, so I used a wheelbarrow. The pile stood eight-feet high, fifteen-feet wide, and fifteen-feet long—enough snow to bury two full-size SUVs.

The digging began at 7:00 a.m. the next morning with a sleepy crew. Matthew, you developed an ingenious digging technique that produced dense blocks of snow, which we used to build a six-foot-high corridor around half the fort and a brick-like castle façade.

The temperature was below zero, which was great for building, but not for nine-year-olds' morale.

By the end of day three, the sight was impressive enough to stop traffic in the street. But the chill and the workload had sapped the spirit of my once gung ho little troopers.

By day four, it felt as if I were running a Russian gulag. "Come on, boys. We said we were going to do this. I told you it was going to be tough. But it will be worth it!" At fourteen, Matthew, you were my biggest supporter, but even you began to question the wisdom of the project. It was eating away your Christmas break, too.

I spent many hours of those next few days working alone.

When the snow fort was complete, it was a neighborhood spectacle. Kids and adults stopped by and asked for tours of the "two-bedroom bungalow" with two entrances. You all enjoyed a week of celebrity before it was time to return to school.

Days later, we got a call from KARE-11, our local NBC news station, asking to do a story on the snow fort. When that cameraman showed up, you put on your snow gear faster than I had ever seen. The TV appearance was a *huge* "dad moment" for me, because I had always told you hard work pays off—and this time it really had.[2]

Snow fort, like my dad: The decisive demand that everyone fall in line, the fanatical determination to finish what you start, and the excellent results we achieved.

Snow fort, unlike my dad: The very idea of a snow fort; the understanding that you were losing your Christmas break, that it was miserably cold, and that this dream was more mine than yours.

★ ★ ★

It's not lost on me that I'm heavily focused on fathers and sons and discipline here. Nurturing *was* a part of my equation, but it came second to discipline. Plus, I knew Kristin was providing it to you in the same way my mom provided it to me, so I've been less conflicted about that.

I've been much more conflicted about my dad and what kind of dad I wanted to be. He taught me in an imperfect and somewhat

---

2. The news story and photos of the snow fort can be seen at www.tellmysons.com.

unintentional way about what parenting and leadership really is: an example (action) that inspires or deters, encourages or discourages, empowers or disempowers—or, as I've learned in life, a little bit of all the above.

I turned out to be a pretty decent person. *Does that mean my parents had it right?*

You'll meet people in life who were gentler parents but had kids who turned into criminals. *Did those parents have it wrong?*

I've had decades to test, prove, and disprove what I liked and didn't like from my youth. I spent most of my undergraduate work in social studies and teaching, digging into child development, sociology, and psychology. And yet, I still have more questions than answers.

That said, I propose to you that although there are few things in life more complex and uncertain in outcome than child rearing, we do know that some techniques work better than others. We also know that kids get a deciding vote in the equation by way of their personalities and life choices.[3]

In the final analysis, my story is *an acknowledgment* that no father or leader is perfect, but that every father borrows the best of what he's observed and tries his hardest to shit-can the rest. It's my hope that you do the same and that you do it at least as deliberately and carefully as I have.

When I think about my own mixed emotions and imperfect memories of my dad, I do wonder what you all will remember about me. This is a timeless consideration that was best explained by Mark Twain when he quipped, "When I was a boy of fourteen, my father was so ignorant I could hardly stand to have the old man around. But when I got to be twenty-one, I was astonished at how much the old man had learned in seven years."

---

3. One of the best conversational works on the complexities of child rearing I've ever read is David Brooks's *The Social Animal*. I recommend chapters three through nine, which gives a far richer account than what I think about the subject.

Unless there's a cure for cancer, you won't see me when *you* turn twenty-one, and that's the age when I was only beginning to understand the virtue in my dad's actions and words, even if I didn't always adopt them.

As an adult, I was able to see him build his own four-thousand-square-foot home. Working with him on that house provided a hundred tiny clues about a simple wisdom I was blind to in my youth.

For thirty years he worked in construction, and I saw him exercise responsibilities commensurate with an army brigade commander. Despite a healthy pension and a body worn hard by dozens of years working in Minnesota winters, he picked up his tools and went right back to working ten-hour days, for himself.

He heats his home with wood, and he cuts and splits every piece of oak that goes into that furnace, which is no small feat for a northwest Wisconsin home.

I've seen him climb trees with his bare hands and feet, and I've heard about him climbing right back up after falling out of them.

When the fishing is good in late winter, he uses a ladder to cross open water to reach the receding ice.

He's a perfectionist, and his sense of pride is often too much for his ego to handle, but when he takes on a task, you can bet your life it will be done exceptionally well.

When I hear people call him crazy for ignoring a warning or advice about what can't or shouldn't be done, I can only nod in agreement and smile, because I've heard those same words as a cadet, a student teacher, a soldier, an officer, a husband and father, and a cancer survivor.

Our man-to-man experiences helped me temper my immature, youthful memories of him. His "madness" was actually all about taking calculated risks, often choosing a path of difficulty and challenge over comfort, being literally and figuratively willing to walk on thin ice, and relying on actions over words to get things done.

I know your memories of me may be dominated by visions of the same hard hand my dad held over me, and naturally I want you to see virtue in *my* madness. I can only hope my stories about his actions will help you see the wisdom (and feel the love) in mine.

⋆ ⋆ ⋆

Words mean things. Words: mean things. MacArthur didn't say to disregard them; he said to make sure you don't substitute them for action. My experiences in combat and with cancer, and the conversations that resulted, have taught me that too many people seem to think sentiments are strong enough without action. Don't you believe it.

Or as a drill sergeant once told me, hope in one hand . . .

CHAPTER THREE

. . . PROUD AND UNBENDING IN HONEST FAILURE, BUT HUMBLE AND GENTLE IN SUCCESS.

September–November 2010

When the day finally came to leave the hospital on September 8, five weeks after I went in, I felt like a baby bird being pushed from the nest with no feathers on its wings.[4]

I had only been eating solid food for a few days, weighed 130 pounds (down from 165), and could barely walk. Bullah was still a fist-size drainage pocket inside my body, and Buford was still a quarter-inch-wide slit across my abdomen that leaked digestive juice 24/7.

Oh, and I still had cancer.

When we got home, my eyes misted at every turn. Everything was just as I had remembered it, but I was not, and that mismatched

---

4. Medically curious readers may find details for the "how" and "why" of my release from the hospital and other blow-by-blow details in my online CaringBridge journal, www.caringbridge.org/visit/markmweber.

feeling was intense.

I glanced at the massive half-acre garden that had taken me three years of backbreaking labor to create—completed just two months before my cancer diagnosis. Now I was so weak and feeble, I couldn't even trim a rose.

On my way to the bathroom to take a shower, I walked past our bedroom. Intimacy of any kind with my wife would not be possible for the foreseeable future.

I went to take a shower, and I was not at all prepared for what happened. At the hospital, the only thing I ever saw in the small vanity mirror was my face. In our bathroom, we had mirrors large enough to see my body from the waist up. Undressed, I turned to get a towel and caught a full glimpse of my naked body. The sight took my breath away.

I could see every rib in my chest, my shoulder bones jutted out in sharp points, and my arms and legs looked like sticks. My butt was gone, my back just connected to my legs in one seamless line. And I was hunched over like a ninety-year-old man.

What in the hell had I done to myself?

I sat down on the toilet seat and sobbed uncontrollably in deep heaves. The visual reminders of the changes were just too overwhelming. For weeks, I had thought of myself as the same strong, fit, army soldier I'd always been, and I had wondered where this silly pot belly had come from. Now I realized my stomach was about the same size it had always been; the rest of my body had just shriveled around it.

Food selection became an Olympic event: great hope for success, devastation in the frequent failures. And every crap was an emergency.

My body seemed incapable of controlling its temperature: if I pulled on a sheet, I'd wake up soaking wet; if I used nothing, I'd wake up freezing cold. And my bandages could never contain the volume of leaky digestive juices for more than an hour.

For the first time in my life, I experienced night terrors, and they were frequent. I would wake up yelling and thrashing from dreams I could not remember.

Each of these conditions prevented me from sleeping. I was exhausted, but I could never get more than two hours straight. I had to sleep on a twin-size air mattress in our living room—the same one I'd used in Iraq for a year.

For the next three months, we measured success and failure by digestion, weight gain, and bowel movements—and also by my mood, which wasn't quite the same as the jut-jawed army soldier I had so recently been.

After a few weeks, and with the constant sentiment of the Serenity Prayer rolling through my mind, I resolved that I needed to push some boundaries to see what changes I could affect.

I started with the pain medication. Many of my conditions stemmed from the fact that my entire body was half-asleep, yet I still seemed to feel pain. After a brief consult with my doctors, and against their advice, I stopped the meds cold turkey. The all-night drenching sweats, the agony of restless leg syndrome, and an incomprehensible level of nausea made me appreciate the "rebound effect" of any heavy narcotic. On each of the first four, worst days, I seriously considered popping a couple of those pills, but I held out hope, based on others' experience.

Just one more day, I told myself every night. *It will get better.*

In the weeks that followed, my bowels began to move, which improved my mobility and digestion and advanced my healing dramatically. Soon I found I could do useful work around the house, though I liked warning people it would not be wise to pay me by the hour.

I still experienced a lot of pain, but not much more than when I was on the drugs. And I found that a clear head made the pain tolerable. *Tradeoffs.*

Whenever I felt like complaining, I thought about being

stoned, constipated, and thick-headed. The power of that perspective helped me maintain my resolve.

But then on November 2, 2010, a CT scan revealed the remaining cancer had rapidly progressed and was now inoperable. The treatment options were essentially nonexistent. "I think you're looking at March or April"—four or five months—"at the latest," my oncologist told us.

This wasn't supposed to happen. My diagnosis had been a "slow-growing" version of pancreatic cancer. *What the hell happened in three months that it was now going rogue?*

We moved my treatment from the Mayo Clinic to the Virginia Piper Cancer Institute in Minneapolis so I could be closer to home—to die.

I began preparing for my funeral. I wrote to my childhood priest, planned and wrote out a set of funeral details, expressed my final wishes, and even organized the funeral reception. I thought about writing letters to you boys and Kristin, but I already had twenty-two-years' worth of journal entries. *What more could be said?*

At Piper, my newly assembled medical team injected new energy into my treatment. Instead of blank stares and resigning to the diagnosis handed to me at Mayo, they actually listened to what I told them about the inconsistencies in how the cancer was acting. I hadn't gone there for a second medical opinion, but that's what they wanted to give me.

Mayo doctors had dismissed several tests because they didn't think the outcome would change my treatment options for pancreatic cancer. Of course, this would have been true *if I had had pancreatic cancer.*

Three weeks later, on Thanksgiving of all days, pathologists at Piper confirmed with an unmistakable air of giddiness that they had discovered what two previous pathologists at two different hospitals did not: I did *not* have pancreatic cancer, nor did I have any disease even remotely related to the pancreas.

I had gastrointestinal stromal tumor—or GIST, for short. There was still no cure, but the good news was that there were chemo treatments consisting of a lot more than magic beans and hope.

✳ ✳ ✳

At a very early age, I had the chance to taste both exceptionally bitter defeats and the sweetest successes. My dad raced cars. And until I was fourteen, every Friday and Saturday night was filled with adrenaline as we prepared for the excitement of Raceway Park in Shakopee, Minnesota.

In many ways, the emotional ups and downs I experienced later in my life always paled in comparison to watching "Dynamite Denny" race his black, gold-trimmed, '57 Chevy around a quarter-mile asphalt track every summer. It had painted flames on the hood and front fenders, a white-and-red-trimmed "26" emblazoned on the door panels and roof, and slightly canted front tires that helped with steering on the steep banks of each turn.

The deep-throated grumble of that 350-cubic-inch small-block engine with no muffler filled my young senses with a strength and power that seemed supernatural. We knew those races were coming every week, but Dad *always* startled us when he fired up the engine to put it on the trailer for the race. My brothers and I knew nothing of racing outside of Minnesota, so his races may as well have been NASCAR events.

At the track, my brothers and I would head to the back of the grandstand, where two massive trees stood twenty yards apart. After a heated debate over who was going to be number 26, we ran our own twenty-lap "hobby stock" footrace around those trees. Bumping was allowed, but anything too rough would earn a black flag out of the race—a ruling that was self-administered because we were gentlemen, after all.

Two things we always wanted but were never allowed to do: drive with dad to the races and hang out in the pits during the race. At the end of the race, everyone was allowed into the pits, but not knowing what happened during the race gave it a mystical quality. To conjure a feeling of intense anticipation today, I need only remember what it was like waiting for those big wooden doors to open.

One night we approached a chaotic scene in the car stall where my dad parked his truck and trailer. Something was wrong, and tensions were high. A fight? No. Someone badly hurt? Worse. Dad's race car had been "claimed." An arcane and rarely practiced rule of racing in those days said if you won a race, another driver could claim your car for $150. In return, you would get his car, which was presumed to be a piece of shit.

It speaks to the enduring power of human emotion that here and now, some thirty years later, my eyes fill with tears as I recall that day.

My brothers and I quietly sobbed as we watched that son-of-a-bitch Gene Kreuger drive off with our beloved number 26. *Hate* is a strong word, but that's what I felt that night.

And what did we get in exchange? A *pink car* with a plain white "X2" painted on the doors. We were horrified. Not only had we suffered the indignity of having our car taken, but we got an abomination in return.

Dad was stone-faced. He and his crew scoured the pits that night for every can of black spray paint they could find. It was 11:00 p.m., and everyone was tired and ready to go home, but he wasn't leaving those pits until he made that car his.

The next weekend, after seven nights in the garage with his pit crew, he took that car out onto the track and not only beat Gene Kreuger, but won the feature race. There was no boasting or thumbing of noses at Kreuger. The victory alone was enough.

The lesson regarding the failure and success of that experience was all unspoken. The car is important, but it's the skill, attitude, and the determination of the driver and the team that wins the race. Dad never did get his old car back, but only because he didn't want it anymore.

✷ ✷ ✷

Few memories endure like a fist fight. The act touches the nerve root of the human instinct for survival. My first came at Palace Playground in Saint Paul, Minnesota, when I was twelve years old.

Billy Bean was a bully right out of a storybook—long, oily hair; always dirty and unkempt. When we saw Billy, we instinctively went the other way.

If Billy was the stereotypical bully, I was the stereotypical wimp. I knew how to stand up for myself verbally, but if things ever got physical, I walked away, a pattern of behavior that eventually made me a target of bullies.

One day I looked at Billy the wrong way. I didn't need any hints about what to do when he responded with an invitation to fight. I dismounted my tire swing and took a direct line toward home. But Billy followed, taunting me as I walked the long, hundred-yard blacktop path that led straight to the driveway of our home. I was tempted to run, but I remembered Dad said never to run from a predator you can't outrace.

My head was down. I walked with a slump. Despite his taunts to turn and face him, I refused. I was so afraid. My heart felt as if it were in my throat, and I wanted to cry. *Why me?*

About halfway down the path, I lifted my head and saw someone standing in our driveway. It was Grandma Weber. She was holding my baby brother, Charlie, in her arms. She was yelling something to me, but I couldn't make out what she was saying. Come home? Hurry home? She *must* have seen what was going on. Perhaps she had come out to provide some comfort. She was gesturing with one arm as if to gather someone into a hug. Suddenly I caught on. Her gesture was intended as the swing of a fist, and she was saying, "HIT HIM! FIGHT BACK!"

A hot surge of adrenaline made me clench my right hand into a fist. I wheeled and threw the first punch I had ever thrown, straight into Billy's face. The stunned look in his unsuspecting eyes only encouraged me more, and I let loose. His inability to match my effort surprised and emboldened me even more. *I had him!*

Even amidst all that unbridled fury, I wanted only one thing, "Are you going to leave me alone?" I demanded as I held him in a headlock. "I want you to leave me alone! *Never again*, you hear me? Never again!" Pleadingly, he promised.

Billy Bean never came near me again, and I learned a vitally important lesson about how to deal with bullies.

I never did feel good or proud about that fight, but I never once relaxed around him, either. As far as I was concerned, I'd caught Billy Bean on a bad day and gotten lucky. It wouldn't be the last time I felt humility in "victory."

✫ ✫ ✫

With due respect to General MacArthur, *pride in an honest failure* is not always a virtue. I experienced such a moment during a visit to our rustic summer cabins on Crosslake, Minnesota. There was a dustup with my younger brother, Chris, over who would get to sit in the front seat of our family van. I lost the fight as well as my mother's vote when she returned to the van after her shopping. I didn't think I deserved the treatment I got—from a *younger* brother or from my mom.

She told me if I didn't like the decision, I could walk home. *That was fine by me.* As that van drove off, I didn't give the decision a second thought. Instead, I explored my options under a very hot sun.

I had three choices: I could walk the five-mile trek around the cigar-shaped lake, hitchhike a ride, or make the one-mile swim across the lake, none of which I had ever done before. I walked toward the lake just a hundred yards or so away to make a visual assessment of the distance, thinking as I walked, *I'm as good a swimmer as Dad, and he said he swam this distance when he was my age.*

After no more than two minutes of reflection, I convinced myself this was something I always wanted to do, anyway. The trick, I remember my dad saying, was to roll over on your back and float if you ever got tired. Don't panic. Don't think about it. Just swim—nice and easy.

As I walked into the lake with my clothes and shoes on, I was conscious of how peculiar the scene might look if anyone saw me. This was Crosslake's main public beach, which was buoyed off with multiple warning signs regarding the dam that lay fifty yards ahead. But no one took notice.

About a quarter mile out, I stopped to check my progress. This was the longest distance I had ever swum, and our cabins were barely visible in the distance. *Had I made a mistake? Should I turn back now?*

Don't panic. Don't think about it. Just swim.

Halfway across the lake, I found myself heaving pretty hard and again doubting the wisdom of my decision. There was too much time and too little scenery to otherwise occupy my mind. I comforted myself by thinking about the added satisfaction I was going to feel walking up on that shore on the other side. Hopefully my mom and brothers would be there to see it.

I flipped over on my back and rested a few minutes, letting myself bask in the vision. What I heard next as I lay there with my ears underwater shocked me out of my premature pride: the unmistakable sound of a nearby boat motor.

In a flash, I thought about our twenty-year-old neighbor, John, who had been run over by a boat just a few years earlier. He suffered brain damage, permanently slurred speech, and a hobbled walk.

The approaching boat looked as if it were coming straight at me. I began furiously kicking water with my legs and hands in the hopes he would see me. I decided that if my warning signal didn't work, I would need to be prepared to dive and swim as deep and as hard as I could.

That boat ended up passing a solid hundred yards away, and the driver didn't even seem to notice me, but I had a sudden sense of urgency about getting off that lake.

At about that same time, someone at the Weber cabins took notice. "Do you see that person way out there? Some moron is swimming in the middle of the lake!" When no one could find me along the road where they last saw me, my family concluded the moron in the lake must be me. A boat was sent out for me, but I refused it. My original decision may have been born out of laziness regarding the five-mile walk, but I hadn't come this far to be rescued by a boat.

When I reached the shore and tried to stand, my legs felt like rubber, and I could barely walk. I felt proud, but the family video will show I was humble in my victory. I looked like I expected an ass-chewing from my dad. Instead he greeted me with a smile, a firm handshake, and a congratulatory remark. "That took real guts!"

My mom later told me she was proud, too, but more upset about the risk I had taken. "You were going to show me, huh?"

Of course, I had wanted to make a statement about the "unfair" treatment I had received in town, but that message was sent the moment I stepped out of the van. Although I'll never convince anyone otherwise, my swim across the lake was nothing more than a practical decision with an unexpected, but welcome, marker of success.

✷ ✷ ✷

Yesterday's silly argument over who gets the front seat becomes tomorrow's silly argument over leadership styles. I was thirty years old and in command of a 182-soldier military police company at Fort Leonard Wood, Missouri.

It was no secret among most of the senior leaders in our

battalion (my higher headquarters) that our most senior noncommissioned officer (NCO), Sergeant Major Crosby, didn't care for me. He publicly complained I was too involved in soldier care and training, and he took my leadership style as a personal affront to all NCOs. (It didn't help Crosby's ego when my first sergeant rejected his complaints as misplaced.)

When summer came, the battalion held a "unit fun day" that consisted of all sorts of physical challenge events. The culminating event was the "Pugil Pit"—jousting matches with padded sticks used in place of bayonets and rifles.

The ground rules for the Pugil Pit competition were clearly posted on an easel board all day. They were simple: soldiers competed against soldiers, NCOs competed against NCOs, and officers competed against officers. The battalion established such rules to ensure decorum in the ranks.

It came as some surprise, then, when Crosby defied those rules and challenged a senior officer to a fight in front of all our soldiers. That senior officer was me!

My five-foot-eleven, 162-pound frame was hardly a match for Crosby, who carried broad, muscular shoulders, stood six-foot-four, and weighed at least 220 pounds. I hoped someone would cry "foul" at the fact he was violating the rules. But which soldier was going to snuff out an opportunity to watch two superiors pound the crap out of each other? In the pin-drop silence that followed his challenge, I saw no other choice but to accept.

As we donned our protective gear, I tried to remember my hand-to-hand training, and I reassured myself the Pugil Pit was about tactics and techniques, not brute strength. My operations sergeant, Lenny Pabin, was a short, stout, bald firebrand with a strong New England accent. He nervously chatted me up as if he were my boxing cornerman. His words reflected confidence, but his eyes said, "Don't get killed."

Our physical differences were only made more comical as we

entered the makeshift ring, and the voices of encouragement for me were half-hearted and feeble. More soldiers gathered to watch.

Sergeant Major Crosby was a professional, but when I looked into his eyes as we squared off, I only saw one message—"I'm going to beat the living shit out of you, punk."

What happened over the next several minutes was too wild and confusing to describe in any worthy detail, but I do remember the end result: victory and a cheering throng of soldiers for the underdog. I had landed three back-to-back precision kill shots. The match was over in less than ten minutes, and he hadn't made a single point.

I'll admit I felt a strong urge to boast, but I chose a more humble route. Crosby offered a gracious, "Good match, sir, well done," and I replied in kind. It was like fighting Billy Bean all over again. And all over again, it felt good enough just to hope Crosby would leave me alone.

✷ ✷ ✷

Most of the time, good and bad fortunes have a lot to do with hard work, but sometimes dumb luck gets involved. How does a healthy thirty-eight-year-old man who exercises, eats right, doesn't smoke, and hardly ever drinks end up with cancer? It's not fair. But then, I should have died at eighteen.

It was the summer after graduation from high school. My dad pulled into the driveway in a pickup truck loaded to the sideboards with discarded two-by-fours from his construction site. His bringing home that truckload of wood was a summer ritual that resulted in a basement full of cut, split, and stacked firewood for the winter. He left the cutting to me as he departed to finish a roof repair at my grandpa's house.

I laid out the extension cord and went to work with our circular Skilsaw, a heavy-duty, two-handed model with wide carbide tips for a sharper cut.

My dad didn't use a sawhorse, because he said it slowed him down. Instead, he had a technique that allowed him to cut in mid-air. He would hold a piece of wood in his left hand off to his right side and then just lower his saw onto the wood as if he were cutting into a wall. As difficult as this may sound, it was actually much easier, faster, and more efficient than using a sawhorse, so I adopted the practice.

Reach, grab, cut, throw—reach, grab, cut, throw—reach, grab, cut, throw—reach, WHOMP! My momentum was suddenly halted by what felt like a full-throttled punch against the front of my right thigh. At that very instant, I was simultaneously aware of two other senses. First, the sound of the Skilsaw was instantly muted. Second, when I turned to see who punched me, the Skilsaw and my right leg moved as one—as if they were connected.

It took a few seconds to register what had just happened as I looked down at my leg and saw the Skilsaw completely submerged into the flesh. There was no pain, but the blade had cut through my thigh like hot butter and buried itself right down to the femur bone. The muscle tension widened the slit into a red canyon.

I grabbed my leg and pulled the pieces together with my dirty work gloves, hobbled toward the deck to our home's back door, and yelled for my mom. I pulled one glove back and revealed all of that mangled flesh. She didn't even bother with 911. She yelled for my brother Chris and grabbed the car keys. Within seconds, we were on the road *Starsky and Hutch* style—passing cars, jumping curbs, running red lights, my heroically calm mom making her own siren with the horn.

By now the pain was about what you'd imagine after cutting your leg open with a Skilsaw. I bit down on a comb so I wouldn't bite off my tongue.

The only other time in my life I've seen an ER staff move like that was in the movies. The doctor quickly assured us that, despite all appearances, I would not lose my leg. He also said I was one of the luckiest guys he had ever seen. "Another inch to the right or left of that line, and you probably never would have made it here, son."

When my dad showed up, he nearly fainted when he saw the damage. That was quite a moment for me—the first time I'd ever seen him demonstrate weakness and fear.

The cut was so deep, it required two layers of stitches—seventy-six in all. And since I had eaten just an hour before, they couldn't knock me out while they cut away on my leg. The plastic surgeon seemed struck silly by how I had managed to avoid cutting any major arteries or veins.

I was later told a wood splinter had prevented the blade guard from doing its job. When I had leaned over to pick up a new piece of word, the free-spinning blade just *touched* my jeans and pulled itself into my leg in an instant and with little more than one rotation. Had my finger been on the trigger, that blade would have pulled itself into the bone and down through my knee.

So the same dumb luck that gave me cancer had already given me twenty more years and a beautiful family.

☆ ☆ ☆

Victories and losses in life are often a muddled mass of earned and unearned ups and deserved and undeserved downs, with both obvious and mysterious causes.

The first of these experiences was during basic training. In the final weeks leading up to graduation, all talk turned to something called "honor graduates." The best soldiers would compete to earn the title of platoon honor graduates, and the best soldier from all of those would be the distinguished honor graduate for the entire company. Based on my performance, I thought I would at least be a competitor, but my academic work had come up short.

A few days after my non-selection, I was called down to the company orderly room. Drill Sergeant Paradeis sat on a small table outside and stopped me short of the door. "Weber," he said, "you're gonna represent our platoon in the honor grad competition. You up to it?"

"Yes, drill sergeant!"

When I returned to our troop bay, I found out the reason for the unexpected honor. Specialist Miller, one of our platoon's competitors, had been on cleaning detail the night before and got caught with his hand in the cookie jar—*literally*, eating cookies out of the commander's desk.

My late selection put me at a significant disadvantage. The other competitors had days to prepare. I had one night. When I appeared in front of that selection board, I tried to focus on the little things, like the nitpicky formalities required for answering questions. I figured we would all likely know the answers to their questions, but we'd foul up something small and otherwise insignificant.

Unlike the nail-biters we're used to seeing on TV, military announcements don't come with much drama. The first sergeant read through the list in short order, from the top, "The distinguished honor graduate for Charlie Company, 40th MP Battalion, is Private First Class Mark Weber."

For the first time in my life, I had not only accomplished something beyond what I'd thought was possible, but I had come from behind and done it with an exclamation point. I learned later that my victory was the result of a single point on the score sheet from one of those "little things": I was the only soldier to hold my hand salute until my superior lowered his.

★ ★ ★

Four years after basic training, I was a successful airborne paratrooper, a decorated enlisted soldier, and an honor graduate from the army's basic course for NCOs. I went on to complete army officer training amidst a dizzying array of accolades and honors. I graduated at the top of my ROTC class and was one of 250 cadets out of 6,000 to receive the army's General George C. Marshall

Leadership Award.

But nestled right in there with these mindboggling victories was an equally numbing defeat as a student teacher that offset the glowing affirmation and vote of confidence from the training classroom. More about that later.

✫ ✫ ✫

Despite my lackluster performance at Cretin-Derham Hall, Minnesota State University admitted me on a probationary status. With focus and hard work, I graduated four years later with honors. Nine months after that, I graduated as an honor graduate and second in my class of forty at the MP officer basic course. I also won a scarce and highly coveted training seat to the US Army Ranger School.

But within a week at ranger school, I departed with my head hanging in shame after washing out. The torn meniscus in my left knee was little comfort, because I knew a truth no one else knew: I had sustained the injury *prior* to the start of the course. I was disappointed about failing, but devastated by the reason: I had been dishonest with myself. This was a personal and professional embarrassment I could have prevented, but I had allowed pride to blind me.

✫ ✫ ✫

My *personal* failings at ranger school were nothing compared to what I would face just a few weeks later. Assuming command of the thirty-two soldiers of Fourth Platoon, 555th MP Company in November 1994 was like Christmas morning. Eight years of training as a soldier and officer had culminated in this day, and what I received was the equivalent of a bag of coal in my stocking.

If you're looking for a story about a new platoon leader who inherits a mess and turns it all around, you should skip this section, because it isn't here.

The 555th, also known as the "Triple Nickel," had just returned from a grueling thirty-five-day mission in Haiti following a military coup that was falling apart. During their mission, logistical support had been virtually nonexistent, because US forces required more time to get established. Showers came largely from the sky or from rain gutters, food consisted solely of prepackaged meals (MREs), and soldiers had to burn their human waste every day. None of this was backbreaking, however; soldiers train for conditions like this.

What made things uniquely difficult for the Nickel was that they had been sent home early from Haiti. Their mission was seemingly incomplete, and the reasons for the early departure were unclear. Questions about poor leadership only added to the rumors that inevitably followed.

So the soldiers of the Nickel experienced the most emotionally challenging parts of a deployment, but none of the gratification that comes from successfully completing the assigned mission. They had a lot to be cranky about, and they wore their bad attitudes like body armor.

Two weeks after the Nickel's return, the Fourth Platoon was met by a wide-eyed and eager second lieutenant named Mark Weber whose reputation preceded him: "a former National Guard enlisted soldier who failed out of ranger school."

If I was overeager (and no doubt I was), my newly acquired platoon was nearly unconscious. The platoon sergeant, the backbone of the platoon and the "right arm" for *any* platoon leader, didn't even show during my first week on the job. Not even a phone call. The treatment was discouraging, but I was reassured by my predecessor. "He's the best of the best," he told me, "and he knows how to run this platoon blindfolded."

Sergeant First Class Dennis Bryer was a lean, fit, twenty-year veteran, but his gray hair and weathered face suggested a far older man. He had the swagger of someone who knew what he was doing. So instead of dwelling on his absence, I jumped in and got to know the soldiers of the platoon.

With pen and paper in hand, I sat down with each soldier, listened intently, and found myself recoiling in ever-increasing shock. They were unmotivated, depressed, and angry—*at everything*.

Their behavior reflected universal signs of indiscipline. Soldiers showed up late to formation. Physical fitness sessions were poorly attended. Soldiers and leaders came and went as they pleased during the duty day. Because of Haiti, senior leaders seemed either indifferent or entitled. I understood the importance of providing liberal "soldier time" following deployments, but theirs was a free-for-all. Still, I wasn't going to be the self-righteous new guy.

In mid-December, after about thirty days on the job, I informally addressed the entire platoon with all the enthusiasm and passion I could muster, telling them to enjoy a well-earned break with their families and to come back in January refreshed and ready to train hard. That enthusiasm was met with blank stares and silence.

Months later, I learned my remarks were received with abject scorn. These soldiers were universally miserable, and my doe-eyed enthusiasm only reinforced that feeling.

January came fast, and the energy of the platoon dwindled even more, with Bryer setting the dismal tone through his indifference and inaction. We spoke about it, but I always tiptoed, desperately afraid I would commit the cardinal sin of being the new lieutenant who pissed off his more-experienced platoon sergeant.

I was failing. There were good reasons for all of it, but no excuses.

I knew we needed a good team-training exercise where we could all experience and overcome some common hardships together. But the earliest opportunity would be mid-March—too long, in my mind. It wasn't much, but that's where I focused my efforts and motivation.

When March finally came, my anticipation was as strong as it had been back in November when I first arrived. A few days before execution, however, our company commander casually announced plans to use my platoon for company-level training instead.

I pleaded with the commander, telling her I had not experienced a single day of training with my platoon since arriving five months prior. *How about some time to work with them, to ascertain the strengths and weaknesses of my subordinate leaders?* She would not budge, and I hated her for it.

That same day, Bryer told me he wouldn't be able to attend our now-shredded training cycle. He said he needed to attend a training conference in California as a *volunteer* for the Red Cross, and his delivery was just as casual as the commander's notification. Worse, he hadn't come to me, his boss, for the permission he required; he'd gone to the commander instead.

Every person has his limits. I had reached mine. I had already tried positive thinking and motivational speeches. Now it was time for fire and brimstone. I intended to make sure some china got kicked off the walls.

"We need to talk," I told Bryer as I closed the doors to our office. I sat down across from him and leaned forward on my knees. "You gotta tell me what the fuck is going on here, man . . . you gotta come clean. I don't think I've got all the answers here, but I know I'm not a failure, and this *feels* like failure."

His face turned red, and he squirmed in his chair as I bluntly laid out my observations—his constant absences; his college classes and volunteer efforts without my knowledge or approval; and worst of all, his refusal to maintain good order and discipline with the soldiers of our platoon.

Bryer opened with a defense, but it was half-hearted. Suddenly his tone changed, and he offered a candid admission, "Look, sir, here's the deal. You're a good lieutenant. Your skills and your enthusiasm . . . I'm supposed to be that guy. I know I'm supposed to be doing it, but since you've been so eager to do it, I figured I would take care of myself for a change." I sat silent and stunned as he explained that after more than two years on the job, he was just plain burned out.

Bryer's dreadful admission came as a welcome view of truth in contrast to the weekly sense of foggy failure I'd felt for five months. There's no magical ending to my first six months—or my next year—as a platoon leader. Bryer didn't get any better, but his candor about the situation fueled the confidence I needed to remain proud and unbending with my passion and leadership, despite the failures that continued to follow.

★ ★ ★

The failures I endured with Bryer and the Fourth Platoon came with no personal risks, little professional harm, and included only soldiers. A few years later when I was a detachment commander for the 795th MP Battalion, I found myself in a mess that included a soldier's family member. This added a whole new level of complexity, and it posed significant personal and professional risk and harm.

Staff Sergeant Ben Kramer was an excellent administrative NCO—quiet, unassuming, and competent. Unfortunately, he had a spouse who was batshit crazy.

There's no law against being absentminded, unstable, or prone to incoherent fits, but the marital strife was affecting Kramer's work. His wife wasn't paying bills, and when she decided to spray paint the walls of their rented home, their landlord wanted to take legal action.

In the army, such circumstances require the attention of the commander, and that meant far more involvement in the Kramers' lives than any of us wanted. The Kramers were eventually evicted, which required them to move into army housing and brought even more stress and need for supervision. This drama went on for ten solid months, and there was one incident or another at least every other week.

One afternoon, I received a phone call from Mrs. Kramer—a first for her. Frantic and nearly incoherent, she sounded as if she were completely out of her mind about her husband, the house, and their three-year-old son. Before I said a word, the phone went dead. I called back, and their three-year-old son answered. He played with the phone for a minute or two, then hung up. I called again, but there was no answer. I couldn't find SSG Kramer, and I didn't want to overreact by calling the MPs, so I immediately jumped in my car and drove to their house.

No one answered when I knocked and rang the doorbell. I scurried from window to window, which offered a clear view of nearly all of the small, single-story home. I saw a lit candle in the living room and the toddler in a back room, but I did not see Mrs. Kramer. For fifteen minutes, I knocked at the door and rang the doorbell, and I began to conclude she had abandoned the house— or worse.

I found an open window and called out for Mrs. Kramer several times, but there was no answer. When a neighbor came over and confirmed the family trouble, I decided to crawl in through the waist-high window to investigate. I walked over and picked up the toddler, and suddenly there she was standing in front of me—wide eyed, enraged, and stoned senseless.

"What are you doing in my house?" she mumbled. "How . . . how did you get in here?"

I explained myself, told her I was concerned for the child, and then left in a flash.

In hindsight, I'm not sure I would have done anything different, given the conditions I perceived and the instincts I felt *in that moment*. What I knew then was that I was concerned about that kid, period. I did not think about my career. I did not think about my safety. I did what I thought was right with the information I had, and I felt confident my reasonable suspicion of a serious problem would legally cover my rear end.

My boss saw it differently and issued a written memorandum of counseling that informed me that my judgment was deeply flawed. As it turned out, I never was in danger of suffering any permanent damage to my career, but I had no such assurance at the time.

☆ ☆ ☆

Just as failure is sometimes out of your control, sometimes success stems from the most unlikely causes.

In 1998 when I was a senior first lieutenant, I gained the attention of senior colonels and generals across Fort McClellan, Alabama. Did I overcome some incredible obstacle? No. Did I lead a team to improbable victory? No. Had I achieved some amazing standard of hard work and competence? Well, kind of, but not the sort I ever thought would garner accolades. What was the act that earned an inordinate amount of praise? Marching.

In the spring of 1998, army leaders at Fort McClellan were looking for an adjutant to serve during a large military parade. The adjutant is usually the most junior officer in such pageantry, and the job demands a mastery of drill and ceremony that many *career* officers find intimidating. From the spectators to the troops on the field, all eyes are fixed upon this lone actor to get it all precisely right.

Getting selected for such a task was therefore hardly an achievement for me. No one wanted the job. But I did. I'd been marching since I was fourteen, and I knew the painfully long sequence of commands and marches so well, I didn't even need to review a script.

The most embarrassing, undignified, yet impressive task the adjutant must perform on the parade ground is affectionately referred to as "the duck walk." That's what the adjutant looks like during the brisk march he must execute to reach his position on the parade field before the marching formation reaches its position on the parade field.

Nearly every officer I ran into that day—from superiors to

peers to subordinates—commented they had never seen anything so bizarre and impressive at the same time. "Your legs were moving so fast, it looked like you were floating!" One colonel remarked somewhat backhandedly, "That was amazing. You looked like you had a hot fire poker shoved up your ass."

Being exceptionally good at such a "little thing" did not earn me a challenging assignment, a stellar evaluation, or any awards, but it did attract attention to the hard work I was already doing. The career-changing assignment followed months later, and my performance in that job led to the improbable string of successes I mentioned at the beginning of this book.

✬ ✬ ✬

There are certainly enough stories here so far to underscore MacArthur's suggestions on how to balance failure and success. As you can see, I seemed to bounce back and forth between them. Routine failures helped me stay humble in success. And my successes gave me the confidence to be proud and unbending in my honest failures.

But what happens when you experience too many of one and not enough of the other? I propose to you that confidence and humility become harder to calibrate, and MacArthur's equation becomes much more difficult *yet even more necessary* to undertake.

In my case, success began to outstrip failures by ten to one starting in 2002 when I successfully completed my company command assignment. What I began to struggle with then—a little at first and a lot more ten years down the road—was the significance and deservedness of the recognition that followed. And if I ever fell short on self-doubt, there was an occasional peer in the wings who seemed all-too willing to question how it was all possible.

In my twenty-four months of leading a company, I had experienced enough adversity, adventure, and drama to fill a nice-size book. By far the greatest challenge was managing four different deployments to Honduras, Qatar, and Saudi Arabia, while managing training and operations for all of my nondeployed soldiers at Fort Leonard Wood. And then, just halfway through the assignment, terrorists crashed two planes into the World Trade Centers and one into the Pentagon.

Years later, my first sergeant, Joe Vroman, reached out to me and wrote about how impressed he was with my performance during those seemingly impossible times. Seeking perspective and suspect of romantic sentimentality, I pressed him. "What is it that I did that impressed you so much?" His reply is a trophy I cherish:

I recall that when you planned any training exercise or deployment . . . you would always pack so much into the allotted timeframe that I would question (in my own mind) whether we could actually accomplish everything. You would take 30 days' worth of training events and somehow pack it into a 7-day exercise. I used to think you were crazy, but we always got it accomplished with great results!

. . . It may have required longer hours, or focusing on doing the task the right way the first time . . . but either way, we learned to adjust and get it done.

You were hard-nosed and always stuck to your guns . . . always reassuring us that we could accomplish the mission, and it worked (and believe me, I remember leaders coming to me asking for help to change your mind). Whatever the circumstances, we always persevered and came out on top. We never failed to accomplish anything you set in front of us and we became "believers" because of it.

Your constant pushing, and challenging, and questioning, and training, really made the leaders under you learn very quickly to manage their time wisely. It really was inspiring though, because I remember many times coming back from a training exercise with you and sitting in my office going . . . wow . . . did we just do that?

Joe added that I had also helped him personally.

I've never had anyone challenge me to go further, do more, be better, and squeeze more into every day than you did. You taught me to set my sights higher than I ever imagined, and that through hard work, dedication and immense training, we could accomplish anything!

I owe many of my successes in life to you and your mentorship. Although it was completely exhausting to work for you, I can honestly say it was inspirational.

As flattering as Joe's comments were, they highlighted the paradox of successfully pulling off nearly impossible tasks. As he said, many of my subordinate leaders thought I pushed them too hard. I wasn't exactly excited or proud that I was viewed as a slave driver, regardless of how necessary it was. This is the condition that often makes *real* leadership a lonely, depressing position.

It's one thing to do a good job, but it's quite another to do well by others. This philosophy is what drove my every effort in command.

Was it even possible to know if they perceived how truly important this was to me? How could I really know if I made an impact with them?

I knew leaders who reviewed their awards and evaluations as proof, but I learned years earlier never to rely on your own press. How could I separate true appreciation from polite conversation? I remembered how all those trainees heaped praise upon that overweight lieutenant in basic training, knowing full well they thought less.

These questions about effective leadership are like the ones I posed earlier with effective parenting—*we know some techniques work better than others, but the outcome is inherently unknown because of the number of variables involved.*

Three months after I left command, I received an unexpected answer to my collective questions that was difficult to reconcile. I was told that Vroman and the senior leaders of my old company had joined an effort to nominate me for the General Douglas MacArthur Leadership Award, one of the most prestigious individual awards an army officer can receive.

Every year the army selects thirteen active duty officers from an eligible pool of more than thirty-seven thousand officers in the ranks of lieutenant and captain. It is intended to recognize those officers whose work best represents the ideals of General Douglas MacArthur: *duty, honor, and country.*

Officers are measured by their demonstrated leadership and influence, teamwork, physical fitness, adherence to values, proficiency in technical and tactical skills, as well as by less tangible skills like quality of the leadership climate, ability to gain consensus among diverse groups, and achievements that demonstrate an understanding of human nature.

Nominations proceed through several levels of command, and only select files make it to each next level. In fact, there are so many nominees and so many levels of participation, it's wise to just feel honored for being nominated. That's certainly how I felt about it.

But actually winning it?

Four months later, I learned I had. Kristin and I would be flown to a ceremony in Washington, DC, hosted by the chief of staff of the army and the sergeant major of the army.

Within a week, I received another call from Washington. In a completely separate officer selection board, I was told I had been selected as one of twenty captains to participate in a prestigious and rigorous multiyear army program. It consisted of a three-year assignment in Washington, DC, with a one-year sabbatical to complete a fully funded master's program in policy management at Georgetown University, a one-year assignment working on the joint staff of the Pentagon, and another one-year assignment working on the army staff in the Pentagon.

As if all the above weren't amazing enough, just three months later, I received word that a *third* officer selection board had chosen me for "below-the-zone" (early) promotion to the rank of major— one of only two given to MP officers in the entire army that year.

With all that praise and recognition, it was difficult keeping perspective. Even though the affirmation had come from more than sixty independent senior officer assessments on three different selection boards, I knew I personally couldn't be *that* good. This observation forced me to do some heavy reflecting about how to accept praise with the proper amount of humility—and to ask myself what being humble really meant.

I had seen too many people declare they didn't deserve the recognition they received. I considered this false modesty and even the equivalent of a lie. Of course, they deserved some of the recognition, just not all of it.

Real modesty and humility, I thought, *needed to be about figuring out which part of the recognition belonged to me and which part belonged to my team, my peers, and my superiors.*

In the final analysis of failure and success, it may be difficult to tell which is which. I know people who would consider some of my victories to be thinly veiled defeats covered in lipstick.

There's a word for how to see the difference, I suppose: *perspective*. It doesn't come easy, and it doesn't come quick. But it does come if you seek it out or choose to acknowledge it when it is provided.

My dad and brothers acknowledged such perspective in hindsight. Back in the late-1970s, as we stood in the pits at Raceway Park and mourned what I then considered the greatest defeat in my short life, none of us, not even my dad, knew the irony of the story behind that car he "inherited" that night.

Gene Krueger's pink "X2" car was *actually* an intentional throwback to the one driven by nineteen-year-old Dale Earnhardt ten years earlier.

Although Earnhardt became famous driving his number 3 black car, his first dirt-track car was a 1956 *pink* Ford that was branded with a "K2." Earnhardt and his crew intended to paint the car avocado green, but a paint mishap resulted in the car being pink. They couldn't afford to repaint it, so Earnhardt, who would become a *legend* in NASCAR racing and in the houses of Weber, ended up cutting his teeth on dirt tracks in a pink car.

It took us ten years to learn a truth that would have made us reconsider the definitions of success and failure back in those pits. Too late to spare the heartbreak, but in time to give our family a feeling of connection with one of our heroes.

* * *

Honest *failures. Success with* humility.

From black spray paint on a race car, to a single hand-salute, to duck-walk marches, to just a little more care in handling, to managing bowel movements, I have seen that the "little things" mean more than we may know. In fact, I propose to you that doing an extraordinary job with ordinary work prepares you to better tackle the difficult and the complex.

For years, I've hunted down and collected lists of tips—top-ten this and six steps to that—*I hoped could help me avoid failures and achieve success. Those lists are valuable summaries, and you'll find my favorites tucked away on my bookshelf to be read when the spirit moves you.*

But what is just as important as those lists of tips is the value of noticing and caring about what is right in front of your face—simple, common social graces. Please and thank you, *for starters, but also giving credit to others when and where credit is due, taking a personal interest in those you serve or who serve you, and "unplugging" from gadgets and the churn around you in order to give a person your full attention. These are simple to talk about but harder to do, and they not only lead to success, but they also encourage others to help you succeed or manage your failures.*

So an honest failure is one that comes (and will come) *only after a decent attempt at gathering facts, thoughtful consideration toward those who have gone before, and then an honest and objective self-reflection. And success with humility comes* (and will come) *not by trying to be the best, but by doing your best every time and letting the results speak for themselves—to others and to you.*

CHAPTER FOUR

. . . TO SEEK OUT AND EXPERIENCE A VIGOR
OF THE EMOTIONS, A FRESHNESS OF THE DEEP
SPRINGS OF LIFE, AN APPETITE FOR ADVENTURE
OVER LOVE OF EASE.

January 2011

My cancer treatment—a daily oral chemo called Gleevec—seemed to start working immediately. It slowed the cancer's growth, and I was told to be patient and hope for the best. There were GIST patients who got ten more years out of this single medication; others got less than one.

I didn't dwell long on the confusing mix of information or the fact that it was going to take a year or more to recover from the surgical complications. I started exercising more, got my weight back up to about 150 pounds, and let myself believe I was going to get at least two years or more from the Gleevec. I also decided that, despite the slow-growing cancer, I would to try to return to my full-time job with the army as soon as I felt well enough to do so.

"But why? Why not take this time and spend it with your wife and children instead of going back to work?"

My answer was simple then (and remains unchanged): because being an army officer, or being otherwise hard at work, is the closest thing to normal we all know. I didn't know anything about tomorrow, but today I looked forward to the familiar feeling of coming home after a long day at work, having been gone just long enough to miss you and getting to see you all again. In fact, being home all the time felt *abnormal*—to all of us—and it resulted in added stress.

Kristin was not used to my constant presence. It was as if we had been suddenly thrust into involuntary retirement. Without the churn of work to consume my energies, I turned to the environment around me. I could make runs to the grocery store, help with dinner, and organize things in the house. That's when things got bumpy.

Helping out is one thing, but I tackled home duties as the army officer I was—in dire need of a campaign plan. I cleaned out the fridge and freezer, organized the pantry, laid out a meal chart, started tasking you boys with more chores, and proposed ideas to "streamline operations."

Big mistake.

Upkeep of home life was Kristin's domain, and it didn't matter that she sometimes hated doing it. Her dislike of the daily grind of housework was not an invitation for me to take over. As much as she appreciated the help, housework was normal and familiar to her, and they were habits she wanted to keep.

Right around Christmas, we got into a heated argument—our first in more than six months. She kept picking at me, which told me she was itching for a fight. Within minutes, we were yelling and cursing about anything and everything. I think we both knew our anger and frustration had little to do with the subject that started it all, but we raged on all the same. Then it just stopped.

I was out of breath and lightheaded. She came in and sat next to me then broke into a soft cry.

"I'm sorry, Pookie," she said as she leaned on my shoulder. "I like seeing you feisty like your old self. It helps me see you're still in there."

You boys were not spared the "benefit" of my constant presence, either. I knew shared hardship brought cohesion and teamwork, so I looked for ways you could be involved in my treatment and recovery. We settled on the routine task of cleaning out my bile-collection containers. That was nasty work, and just like a trio of soldiers, you couldn't resist bragging a bit about this grim daily drama.

The downside of this "teamwork" was being greeted by a ball-busting army lieutenant colonel when you walked in the door from school. I wasn't a slave driver, but I made sure you didn't plop yourselves in front of the TV.

"Will you ever be going back to work, Dad?" you politely asked, more than once.

✳ ✳ ✳

Based on its title, you might think this book is solely about being a man, a father, and a soldier. Not entirely. This is also a story about being a lover and a husband. It's about the rigors of married life—complicated by the trials of army life and the tribulations of cancer treatment—between two true individuals. In fact, no other experience in my life so completely captures the essence of MacArthur's words on living an emotionally vigorous life.

On July 22, 2010, as we sat in the waiting room at the Mayo Clinic, absorbing the complexities and breathless uncertainties of the journey with cancer in front of us, I became aware that my wedding ring was missing. Even after 16 years of marriage, putting on that ring was a very deliberate, symbolic act every single day. But after the hustle of our 5:00 a.m. start, now I couldn't remember if I had put it on my finger that morning.

Certainly on this day, of all days, I should remember whether I had put on my wedding ring, right?

I couldn't remember.

I also couldn't shake the fear that I did put it that morning but then lost it during the day. It wasn't likely—the ring had never fallen off my finger before. But then again, I *was* down ten pounds from the cancer, and if I *had* lost the ring, looking for it right then and there was the only chance of finding it. I retraced my steps in the few hours we'd been at Mayo. There was really only one place it could have fallen off—the bathroom.

I quietly told Kristin's dad, Ed, about my nagging suspicions. Fellow men of action, we walked straight into that bathroom and started emptying both trash bins of their paper towels—gently unfolding each nasty, damp towel. The bins were filled to the top, so it took a while, but as soon as we approached the bottom, there was a *plink* sound from Ed's bin. We froze and gave each other a quick glance as Ed reached in and pulled my ring from the bin.

I wanted to cry.

Like so many times in our marriage, what seemed lost was found again with an *instinct toward just a little more care and effort*.

We have known each other for nineteen years now. In too many ways, a "successful" marriage between us still seems improbable. We're both fiercely independent, with vastly different tastes and temperaments, and nothing about our lives together has *ever* been routine. Neither of us is certain that we're reflective of a "strong" marriage. But our very survival of the difficulties of army life, infertility, deployments, and cancer must be an indication that we've done something worthy of taking note.

☆ ☆ ☆

To understand the depth of my feelings for Kristin, it is helpful to know the order-loving personality who fell in love with her.

By the time I finally took an interest in women around age nine-teen—I was curious during my teenage years, but more repelled by the work and drama girls seemed to entail—my ideas on romance could arguably be described as fussy and excessively respectable. Of course, I prefer the words *romantic* and *old-fashioned*, but let's not split hairs.

I didn't believe in kissing on the first date, and I disapproved of one-night stands. I was overly sentimental in my affections, and I had a deep conviction about commitment that would find few harbors in the under-twenty-five crowd—then or now.

My first kiss came from a random girl on a dance floor at a club my brother, Mike, dragged me to when I came home for a visit from college. She had too much to drink and reeked of cigarettes. So much for "excessively respectable."

Jenny, my first *real* date and kiss and first relationship, happened a year later, when I was twenty. After a brief romance of maybe a month or two, she told me something I would get used to hearing from all my female friends, including the three girls (yes, exactly three) I dated between her and Kristin: "You're a guy that girls marry, not date."

Peggy was pretty and had an amazing body, but her personality was way too fast and loose for me, and it must have shown in my behavior. She once asked, "Are you gay or something?"

A year later, I met Kari. She was a dream woman—flawless complexion, striking blue eyes, incredibly toned legs and arms, and an easygoing personality. Three months into that relationship, I passed up an opportunity to have sex, because I thought she'd had too much to drink.

Hours later, she whispered into my ear what was by then an old and familiar tune, "You are a *good* and *decent* man, Mark, and you're going to make the best husband someday." She dumped me within a week for being too serious, but she said something that night I still feel good about: "Thank you for what you did . . . for me."

Of course, the next morning when my roommates heard what (had not) happened, they weighed in on Peggy's question about my sexual orientation.

I don't even remember the name of the next girl I dated. I was still reeling from being rejected—three times—for being a gentleman.

* * *

I met Kristin Coughlin in my fourth year in college in late September 1992. My roommates—all varsity basketball players—returned to our apartment from a local bar one night with women in tow. One of those women was wearing a dark purple leather jacket. It was hideous. But the face and figure of that hazel-eyed brunette made me sit up and take notice. The guys pulled out a deck of cards and began playing.

The girl in purple was clearly not versed in cards, and she was too shy to speak up. I moved up next to her on the couch and shyly asked if she wanted some help. I was immediately taken with her personality. Reserved, but sassy and playful, and she was ready with a candid answer to a direct question.

Our interaction that first night was as common as street traffic on a busy road, and I can't say there were romantic sparks.

But something had happened, because over the next days and weeks, we frequently noticed each other in common areas and talked like old friends. Despite a clear connection and real affection, there was no hugging, kissing, or even long looks.

After a frustrating month of confusion on my part, she finally made it clear she had a boyfriend. As upset as this made me, I was impressed then and still today that she meant to keep her declared commitment to him as "girlfriend," despite her acknowledged incompatibility to him.

Mr. Prissy, meet Ms. Krissy.

It wasn't long—but it seemed long to a lovesick boy—before Kristin "officially" broke up with her boyfriend and began dating me. Almost immediately, she invited me to her family's home in Hastings, Minnesota, during the Christmas break for dinner with her parents.

When I pulled up to their residence, it was dusk, which made it easy to see into their house. In the kitchen window, I could see a big, burly figure that appeared to be her dad—*not wearing a shirt*. Did I mention it was December in Minnesota?

When we entered the kitchen, a very hairy-chested Ed Coughlin was standing in front of the sink with a huge smile on his face, sharpening knives in dramatic fashion. I'm certain the look on my face betrayed my shock, and I'm equally certain that shock was the reaction he was going for.

After dinner, Kristin asked me to drive her around Hastings to look at the Christmas lights. The conversation during our hour-long tour was disjointed. We were both distracted and uneasy. We caught sight of a hilariously tacky nature scene painted across the width of a two-car garage door. We laughed so hard, we parked the car. Then suddenly there was silence and tension again.

"Kristin," I brought myself to say, "would you mind if I kissed you right now?"

"Sure," she replied with a smile.

My heart doubled its pace. I slowly leaned over, paused to look her straight in the eyes, and then, as gently as I could, pressed my lips to hers. It was a long, passionate kiss that felt well past due.

Two months into our courtship, Kristin turned to me in a start, looked straight into my eyes, and said, "You know . . . I think I could live with you forever."

You're a guy that girls marry was no longer a curse. I told her I felt the same way.

Our love wasn't blind. We both saw a clash of tastes, interests, and personalities. Though we shared a passion for work and school, she liked '80s, alternative, and new wave music; I liked classic rock and modern pop. She liked schmaltzy Hallmark movies; I liked tough, gritty, action-packed movies. To make decisions, I insisted on deep thought and long reflection; she preferred gut instinct.

I had concerns about how she was going to do with army life. And she worried a lot about how involved my mom was going to be in our lives.

We argued a lot, even in the beginning.

But we had ideals in common.

In a hundred little ways, she demonstrated integrity, loyalty, trust, dependability, and a sound work ethic. She was honest and fair about her opinions and apologies. She was slow to make friendships, but loathe to break them. At work she didn't think it was right to chatter with friends, and she never called in "sick" when her schedule got too full. And she knew how to say "I'm sorry" without conditions or "buts."

Whatever our disagreements, she had strong character, and that overruled any concern I could imagine.

I had always envisioned kneeling and proposing marriage in grand fashion and in some clever way. Instead, I popped the question over lunch and in between college classes while at the River Hills Mall in Mankato. Then we went and looked at rings together. The only deliberate "romance" on my part was that I did it on Memorial Day.

We settled on a wedding date fifteen months into the future and decided to live with each other until then. Grandpa Garofalo approved: "Better to try the shoes on before you buy them."

But there was an elephant in the honeymoon. It was the army. Despite my explanations, I knew she had little idea what it would be like. And neither of us could predict what life would look like six years down the road when my contractual obligation ended.

★ ★ ★

Few things seem more important to a bride than the particulars of her wedding ceremony, but the army quickly reminded us otherwise. Right up to my commissioning, army life was little more than an idle chatter topic. Now it was real. I was ordered to my initial training as an officer in Alabama, and the dates overlapped our wedding.

As we scrambled to explore new options for the wedding, we discovered that the army compensated separated spouses—to the tune of about $2,000 for the duration of my schooling. We decided to elope, *with the army providing our first wedding gift*. In that decision, I saw another opportunity.

With my orders set for April 10, I proposed to Kristin that we marry on April 7—an intentional gesture on my part to communicate to her that I would, whenever I could, put her before the army.

It felt strange standing up at the altar with just our priest, two witnesses, and God. No room for pretense or family approvals and disagreements. No pomp or circumstance.

The scene provided an unanticipated level of intimacy and sincerity that told us a truth we would learn and relearn in the army: We were alone with our decisions and the outcomes, and we would face an imposing life together, without the families that had carried us so far.

✯ ✯ ✯

Our "official" wedding event—still scheduled for its original weekend—was another foreshadowing of how unpredictable our lives would be.

Kristin planned most of the details while I was in training, and when I flew into the Twin Cities one day before the big ceremony, it was like being dropped into a "hot" combat landing zone. There was no bachelor party, I missed the rehearsal, and I was late for dinner. Add months of pent-up sexual tension, and we had the makings for a nice bonfire in the middle of the living room.

The next morning, as three of the bridesmaids were making their way to the church, a drunken off-duty cop ran a red light and T-boned their vehicle.

The accident was so bad, the bridesmaids were put in neck braces and taken to the ER. We later learned that the first responders hiked their dresses up over their heads while they were being strapped to the gurneys, because they pleaded not to have their dresses wrecked. They were late to the wedding and pretty banged up, but they made it.

There was no honeymoon. No long looks. I was on a plane the next day to return to army training.

We laughed when we later found out our wedding would be one of the last held at St. Boniface Church, which was slated for demolition. We hoped our marriage would fare better.

✫ ✫ ✫

My failure at ranger school a few months later resulted in an unexpected early return to Minnesota from Georgia, and I had new army orders in hand for an immediate report date to Virginia. Unexpected, *and unwelcome*, because it meant Thanksgiving and Christmas with her family would be scrapped. It also meant the dramatic change she long feared was upon her.

Emotions flared.

With six days to pack up and say our goodbyes so we could report to Virginia by the date on my new orders, Kristin was beside herself with grief and anxiety. Things were suddenly moving *way* too fast. Adding to the stress, we opted to take advantage of an army financial incentive to pack up and move ourselves across the country.

The conversations that took place during those six days are hazy, but I know they included a lot of cursing and very raw emotions.

I remember yelling at her, "Why in the hell did you marry me? You *knew* this was coming . . . you've known for a year this was coming! This is the army!"

She yelled just as loud in reply that none of it was fair.

The time and distance of the past five months had left our relationship littered with bits of miscommunication, and the recent frustrations had us both wondering if we had made a big mistake.

Before we knew it, we were standing in her parents' driveway with nothing left to say except goodbye.

To help ease the transition, Kristin had hastily adopted two kittens, and Ed found her a used Mitsubishi Starion sports car in pristine condition. But she was still inconsolable. I remember thinking the only time I'd ever seen someone this sad was at a funeral, and the slow procession down the road only added to the effect. Kristin drove my new car, and I drove the moving truck, towing the Mitsubishi on a two-wheeled dolly.

About fifteen miles from Hastings, I passed a driver heading in the opposite direction, frantically pointing to the rear of my truck. I could only hold my head in my hands as smoke poured from under the hood of the Mitsubishi. When Ed and Kristin had loaded it onto the tow dolly, they missed two important facts about the Mitsubishi: it had a *rear-wheel* manual transmission, and it had been left in second gear.

We stopped for the night at the Dollar Inn just south of Chicago. Kristin balked at the cues about the quality of the place—a $19.99 room, a fully enclosed plexiglass desk, and a sign that read, "No refunds after five minutes of check-in"—but it was 11:00 p.m., so I insisted we stay.

When we opened the door to our room, we were transported back in time to the set of a 1970s porno movie. The carpet was a deep shag of reddish-orange, the bed was sunken and had a visible piece of plywood under the mattress, and the air was filled with an undeniable smell of "funk."

All the emotion of the day—*of the week*—was released in a torrent. Curse words flew, and the scene ended with me childishly throwing my wedding band at her as she stormed out the door. Kristin's mom, Karen, still recalls the phone call that came that night: "Mom, I think I made a mistake . . . I want you to come get me." She didn't come.

Kristin returned to the room an hour later, her eyes still red from crying. We made peace, but it felt more like a temporary truce meant only to allow the battlefield to be cleared of dead bodies before the next fight.

The night brought no relief. She insisted on bringing her two kittens into the room, then let them roam instead of keeping them in their carrier. They meowed incessantly, climbed up onto the bed to play, and twisted themselves into Kristin's hair and my face. By 3:00 a.m., they were being tossed across the room like obscenities and wedding rings.

The next morning, we got ready and loaded our things without saying a word. Within minutes of being on the road, we hit an obstacle that was nowhere in our planning for the trip: Toll roads. I had no cash. It was long before mobile phones, and Kristin was too far ahead for me to signal for her help.

"Honey," the attendant told me with a mixture of pity and contempt, "we don't take no checks."

"Well," I replied, "a check is all I've got. Ya see, I'm a moron, and I don't have any cash."

Uncharmed, she took my $1 check. The same scene would play out twice more before we finally stopped for gas.

In hopes of changing our luck, I pointed at the car on the dolly we had destroyed the day before. "Want to see if she still runs?" I asked.

Kristin smiled, for the first time in two days. It took me a while to figure out how to unhook everything, but we finally got the car off the dolly, and it seemed to run okay. (But we would find out later that the engine was blown.) Encouraged, we loaded it back up and drove across the freeway overpass to "Grandma's Kitchen."

We had a breakfast so cheerful that I actually strutted out into the parking lot to get back on the road.

But then my hands moved with ever-increasing tempo from pocket to pocket on coat and pants in search of the keys. My heart sank as I approached the cab of our moving truck. From the ignition they hung, glimmering in the early-afternoon sun.

I found a metal hanger in my trunk and popped the lock open, but the victory was short lived.

As we departed the parking lot, I checked my side mirror while entering the highway on-ramp and saw a shower of sparks flying from the rear of my truck. I had failed to tighten down the safety latch on the hitch, and it had popped off the truck. The only thing that kept the dolly and Mitsubishi from careening into the ditch was the safety chains.

By some miracle, we finally made it to Fort Lee, Virginia, utterly exhausted.

At 6:00 a.m. on our first morning in the army together, we were jolted awake by the sound of a canon blast, followed by a trumpet echo of "Reveille" booming through Fort Lee's loud speakers. I leaned over to Kristin, kissed her on the cheek, and whispered, "Welcome to the army, honey."

"Hmmph," she snorted. "I ain't puttin' up with that bullshit every morning," she said as she snuggled in closer to me.

She would end up putting up with a lot worse than that during our life together—but we'd always become closer in the end.

✬ ✬ ✬

Kristin's birth into army life was a hard labor, but she quickly established who she was going to be and what she was going to do. She had no patience for rank, position, or pomp among army spouses, so she quickly ran afoul of those spouses who did.

She was *not* "the Lieutenant's Wife."

"I have a name," she'd say. "It's Kristin." Military functions were something she begrudgingly attended. One of her common refrains was, "Loving you does *not* mean I need to love or even like the army."

For Kristin, the army was something to be tolerated for about five years until we returned to Minnesota. And if her antipathy toward army life upset the lifers' spouses, it drew younger soldiers' wives to her, because so many of them felt the same way.

One issue we weren't conflicted about was having kids. "What do you think? Time for a baby?" went the conversation. "Sure, let's have a baby."

It was that easy. Matthew, you were born exactly nine months later—one year into our first army tour.

✷ ✷ ✷

Kristin's constant companions during my many long absences were those two cats she adopted, Max and Casey. She loved them *just as much* as you boys love your pets. Back then, this was another source of friction in our marriage. Even with a cat box, I thought they smelled, and I was determined not to have our first home smell like a farm.

What happened next may sound cruel—and Kristin never actually agreed to it—but we kept them outside on our back deck, placed a child-safety gate at the steps, bought a small dog house, put leashes on them, and called it all good. We have an army saying about such ideas: "It briefed well."

It did cross both our minds that our new neighbors—whom we hadn't met yet—might find us odd for treating our cats like dogs. So it wasn't a total surprise the next day when I arrived home ahead of Kristin and found a note taped to the door from our neighbors: "Please come see us when you get this note."

I walked the long driveway to their front door and rang the bell. Three or four kids suddenly appeared in the living room window adjacent to the door and stared at me wide eyed.

Great, I thought, *spectators for the finger-wagging lecture about the proper care of cats.*

"I don't know how to tell you this," my neighbor started, "but I came home from work today and found your cat hanging from your deck. Kind of freaked the kids out, so I took it down." He handed me a covered shoebox, "Here she is. Sorry, man. I'm really sorry."

As I walked the long driveway back to our home, I wondered how I was going to explain this to a pregnant Kristin.

"Honey, I'm sorry, but Casey hung herself off the deck on the leash."

She immediately burst into tears and blurted out, "Dammit, Mark, I *knew* this would happen. You killed my cat!" She beat her fists on my chest but let me hug and hold her as I apologized over and over again for being such a moron. And though my fellow officers still rib me about it seventeen years later, she never gave me grief about it again.

(Until she read the story again in a draft of this book; into the Word document she typed, "dumbass.")

✯ ✯ ✯

Deployments were never far from our minds, because we knew at any moment, long days of field training in the woods could turn into a yearlong absence abroad. We saw our neighbors going through it while raising their newborn, and we both wondered how we would be able to get through such a trial, considering our difficulty just getting across the country together.

My first deployment came when you were only six months old, Matthew. You and I seemed to get along pretty well before I left, but when I returned several months later, it seemed a purple dinosaur named Barney had effectively replaced me as your male role model.

I don't remember a more painful feeling in my life than the one I felt when I reached out to you and you recoiled as if you didn't know who I was. I thought it would get better with the passage of time, but you seemed distant for years after that.

With Kristin, the time apart was difficult, but it was also apparent that separation gave us a greater appreciation for each other.

Although we still bickered about everyday things, like most married couples do—how and what we spent our money on, how we spent our free time, likes and dislikes of life in general—the only issue that seemed to truly plague our relationship was how to manage life in the army.

★ ★ ★

Packing up and moving a house is one of the most stressful experiences a married couple can go through. It's even more stressful when you're a Minnesota couple with army orders to Alabama—a place where "yah" and "you betcha" draw some attention.

Three years earlier, I had to pry Kristin free of Minnesota to go to Virginia. Now the idea of leaving Virginia was just as traumatic and undesirable.

When I got to Alabama in the winter of 1997, I started my job and fell in with a work force (soldiers) that shared the same values, work expectations, and organizational culture as the ones I had just left.

When Kristin got to Alabama, she got "Ya ain't from 'round here, are ya?" One woman approached Kristin after a CPA review course in Birmingham and said in a deep Southern drawl, "Ah just *love* yo British accent."

There was no job waiting for Kristin, and no business interested in hiring someone who was going to leave in two or three years. Fort McClellan's housing was full, so we rented a house in the Alabama countryside. And unlike Virginia, our neighbors were anything but pleasant.

We found out part of the frustration came from the Pentagon's plan to close Fort McClellan. For the local community, which faced a $600-million-per-year economic loss, the news was devastating.

After a few months with no "welcome," Kristin decided to walk to our neighbors and introduce herself. When she rang the doorbell, she saw a quiver of movement in the curtains from a nearby window and awkwardly waited for someone to answer the door. Just as she turned to leave, an angry barking dog come bounding around the corner of the house.

There were no more attempts to reach out to the neighbors.

A year later, our landlords decided to sell their home while they could, forcing us to move. Fortunately, Fort McClellan had *plenty* of empty housing, and we moved into a modest duplex. Unfortunately, because of my job, we'd be one of the last families to leave the post.

When departure time arrived eighteen months later, most of the homes, stores, and buildings were boarded up with plywood. We felt as if we lived in an abandoned city.

✳ ✳ ✳

In 1999, when orders arrived sending us to Fort Leonard Wood, Missouri, we were ready to leave our three years in Alabama in the rearview mirror. The move was our fifth in six years, but this one was particularly stressful—emotionally *and* physically—due to the lack of neighborhood social interaction.

As usual, we chose to move most of our own belongings to take advantage of the financial incentive the army offered. I drove the moving truck, and Kristin drove ahead of me with Matthew in our new Toyota Tacoma pickup truck.

As we crossed into Tennessee after three hours on the road, we both felt ready to stop for the day, but we opted to press on after a quick rest stop.

A half mile down the road, Kristin pulled onto the shoulder, as if she needed to stop. *I wonder what she wants,* I thought.

Just then, her pickup truck veered straight off the road into a long, deep ditch. We were traveling 70 mph. The truck bounced wildly, as if it were about to tip end over end, until it finally plowed into a group of trees. *Oh, dear God, let them be okay, let them be okay, let them be okay.*

When I reached the bottom of the ravine, thirty yards from the road, the scene inside the cab was surreal. Kristin had a white-knuckle grip on the steering wheel, Matthew was whimpering with his blanket over his face, and music—*Disney* music—blared from the radio as smoke streamed out of the air vents.

"Kristin!" I yelled. "Are you okay?!" She had a look of sheer terror on her face. Without waiting for a response, I pulled her out of the truck.

"I fell asleep, and I wrecked your new truck," she finally sobbed while frantically waving her arms. That loud Disney music had been for her, not Matthew. I grabbed her head and held her firm so our eyes were about two inches from each other and quietly told her, "Fuck the truck."

I pulled her into a hug and held her tight, rubbing her back and trying to get her to calm down. "It's going to be okay . . . you're okay . . . Matthew is okay . . . now we gotta get focused here." Within minutes, passersby and a state trooper offered assistance.

As we all pulled away from the scene, I couldn't help but notice the wide *cement* bridge abutment just a couple hundred feet from where Kristin crashed. Things could have been *a lot* worse.

With the loss of the Tacoma, and with a moving truck filled to capacity, we were forced to leave behind all of our house plants, one of which was a spider plant that had been on the wedding altar with us five years earlier. The body shop owner placed everything in a large storage shed.

A month later, we drove back to Tennessee for the repaired truck. When the owner opened the shed, we were stunned at what we saw. All of our plants were brown and dead, except one—*that spider plant.* It was in rough shape, but it had survived. (And it's still alive today.)

★ ★ ★

Next to moving, having kids is a close second for marital stress, and life had given us a leather belt called "infertility" to chew on for a good four years while we were in Alabama and Missouri.

A visit to the doctors in 1998 revealed I was clinically sterile. This diagnosis was our first exposure to the inexact science of medicine we would experience so many years later with the cancer.

"What does *clinically* sterile mean, doc?" I asked. He told me that typically it takes about fifty million sperm to conceive a child, and at least thirty million of which need to be healthy. In my case, there were fewer than one million sperm, and more than 99 percent were either deformed, had no tail, or couldn't swim straight (a metaphor for my life, my friends and I jokingly agreed).

"But," the doc smiled, "it *does* only take one."

At those odds, "trying" unavoidably turned intimacy into a chore.

There was also a miscarriage, which felt like a punch in the teeth. It had been a "blighted ovum" (unfertilized egg mimicking pregnancy). I later joked with Kristin that she was so eager to conceive, she tried to do so without me.

One of the options presented to us was in vitro fertilization. The only thing I remember about that conversation was the $10,000 price tag—*per attempt*. And it would likely require three attempts. We didn't have that kind of money, and the discussion only added to the stress.

In January 2000, we gritted our teeth, signed the paperwork, and began the scheduling process for the procedure. About a week or so later, Kristin commented she was "late." We both half joked about the irony and the possibilities, but I wasted no time running off to fetch a pregnancy test.

Even after the test showed positive, and a blood test confirmed it, we both reflected on our blighted ovum experience.

Nine weeks later, I came home for a quick visit from an army school at Fort Leavenworth and found Kristin lying on the couch crying. She had just come from her first ultrasound. My heart sank. *Not again.*

"Look at the picture," she said with despair dripping from her voice. As I did, my brain truly could not process what I was looking at. There was a hand-drawn circle with a line that led to the words *baby #1*, and then a second circle and line leading to the words *baby #2*.

"Twins?" I asked with tears welling up in my eyes. "My God, we're having *twins*?!" Even more miraculous, we had fertilized *two* separate eggs—fraternal twins, just like my twin brother and me.

"Why on earth are you crying?" I pleaded.

"*Two* babies in *this* little body?" she moaned. "They're going to destroy me. How am I going to be able to handle *twins*?"

Kristin was and still is a five-foot-six, 116-pound frame, and she remembered that you, Matthew, were nearly nine pounds at birth. (Joshua and Noah, you ended up weighing a total of 13 pounds.)

There was no consoling her. And worse, two days later, I had to return to Fort Leavenworth five hours away to complete three more weeks of school.

✫ ✫ ✫

The deadliest and most significant battle of the American Civil War—widely believed to be a pivotal turning point of the American experience—began as a light skirmish between cavalry scouts at a crossroads in a sleepy little town called Gettysburg. Eighty years of unity as a nation somehow failed to prevent 176,000 Americans from converging on that place and killing or wounding more than 50,000 of each other in just three days.

For four months in the spring of 2000, Kristin and I arrived at a similar crossroads, despite our own history of unity. For us, the stakes felt just as high.

Our initial "skirmish" occurred over the issue of obtaining a larger vehicle for our growing family. Kristin felt life was going to be hard enough with Matthew, twins, *and* the army; she refused to struggle with the vehicles we had. For my part, I had no intention of putting us in $35,000 of debt for a vehicle we wanted but didn't need.

The discussion about vehicles naturally shifted to our overall financial stability, which was directly linked to the mother-of-all stressors in our marriage—*leaving the army.*

The occasion for the looming battle was straightforward. My six-year obligation to the army would end in just a few weeks. Our discussions in years prior were usually intense, but never decisive.

In short, leaving the army was going to require finding a new job, looking for a new place to live, and moving, in that order. The pending arrival of newborns meant Kristin wasn't going to work anytime soon, and in all likelihood, I could expect an extensive pay cut *when* I found a job.

I thought Kristin played down these concerns. She thought I exaggerated them.

"I've seen you at work," she said. "This will all be much easier than you're making it seem." Plus, she believed she had held up her end of our unofficial "bargain" regarding length of service. The time had come for me to honor and reciprocate her sacrifice with options closer to *her* ideal.

We threw ourselves into an all-out debate, despite the fact that a six-week army school kept us physically separated. I think we both knew we couldn't kick that can down the road anymore.

Perhaps partly because of the safety of distance, push quickly turned to shove, and punch followed close behind. We knew each other's hot buttons, and we pressed *all* of them in an attempt to sway the other.

All Kristin heard from that point forward was an insincere,

controlling husband who wanted to stay in the army no matter what.

All I heard was an irrational and ungrateful wife who wanted to leave the army no matter what.

The word *divorce* was never uttered, but the language and tone were unmistakable.

For the first time in our lives together, the *true* meaning of love and commitment was being tested for both of us, and strangely, it seemed clear there really wasn't a right answer.

For years, I'd been told that finding a job I truly loved was as critical to a happy life as marrying someone I truly loved. The army wasn't just our stable (and sole) source of income; it had become an incredibly fulfilling life choice for me. *And to my pleasant surprise, I was good at it.*

Leaving the army would mean starting all over in a new culture with no network of coworkers or former bosses. In short, precisely what Kristin had endured for six years, an irony that was somewhat lost on me at the time.

What if Kristin chose not to work after the twins came along? What if leaving the army *didn't* produce her ideal, but instead replaced one set of sacrifices and uncertainties with another? I knew she might resent me if we stayed in the army, but I also knew enough about myself to realize I would resent her if my resignation didn't lead to happiness on her part.

In a matter of days, our fight turned into a dangerous game of chicken. I was cold, mean, and rough—and I meant to be. I told her if her life was so horrible and unfair, she should "pack her shit" and move home. Then I refused her calls and didn't return letters. That was the wrong thing to do to a pregnant woman. She did just what I told her to do.

The months that followed were emotionally brutal. Kristin turned cold, distant, and unresponsive. In a real game of chicken, you can both see each other's car. What we were doing was the equivalent of playing the same deadly game, but with blindfolds on.

Within weeks, I began to seriously question both my judgment *and* her response to it all. How could I treat a pregnant woman this way? And why would she risk losing a decent husband and father with three kids in tow? I also noticed that the answers mattered less and less to me. Instead of looking backward at what had happened or looking for her to change, I started looking at what I was gambling with.

I saw a woman who was tireless as a mother, with volunteer work, and with her pursuit of improving herself professionally despite the lack of a career. In all my days, weeks, and months away from her and our home, her eyes, her heart, and her attentions were always upon me. She was one of the fiercest fighters I'd ever met when she got upset, and in light of her consistency of character, I realized she was a fighter I wanted on my team—*even if I got in the line of fire every once in a while.*

So, were Kristin's hang-ups with the army something to split up over? What was it that I found unreasonable about her resistance to life in the army? That she didn't like moving her home and losing personal contact of all her friends every two or three years? That her dignity was shredded every time she had to quit a good job and try to find another in a community that didn't like hiring army wives? That she didn't like the idea that her husband and the father of her kids could be taken away from home for months or a year at a time with little warning—and maybe not return? Those who have learned to embrace such turmoil and change should be commended, but was it such a crime for her to be so opposed to these things?

My answer to each of these questions was that Kristin's reasoning may not have been fully considered, but it wasn't irrational. I didn't suddenly abandon what I believed were fundamental obstacles in the equation. I just decided that if our little war might cost me Kristin, the army and my ego would have to be casualties instead.

If I was decided on the matter, Kristin certainly was not. My pledge to ditch the army fell on deaf ears. As if to meet my "pack your shit" comment with equally dramatic flair, she remarked, "Well, I think I need some time."

The truth is, she didn't believe me. She thought I was telling her what she wanted to hear, which wasn't such a stretch, considering my passion and devotion to the uniform. Maybe she wanted me to stew in the juices of my convictions for a bit. *How bad do you really want it?*

Our meetings in public places made it feel as if we were legally separated and already sharing child custody. It was so cold and distant, the memory still fills my eyes with tears.

She later admitted that fear drove her every thought and action back then. For six years, she felt she had played second fiddle to the army and, despite evidence to the contrary, had become weaker. If she were overreacting, she felt she had good reason. She had little employment history, no job, and no income.

Absolutely nothing in our lives together justified any of these thoughts, but emotion and a mother's protective instincts had completely trumped reason. The situation became even more complex and devastating when we learned her dad was diagnosed with prostate cancer.

Obviously, our civil war had a happy ending because we're still together. Even her dad's prostate cancer had a happy ending (at the time) following his surgery. But the story gets so much better.

My refocused love and commitment toward her resulted in *her* refocused love and commitment toward me. It was as if she just wanted to know—*with absolute certainty*—that she was more important than the army. Once she had that reassurance, everything else was relatively insignificant.

We started compromising more. Together we worked out never-before-considered options for making army life more tolerable for her. She missed her family terribly. And the most meaningful solution was also the easiest—routine annual visits to

Minnesota just for her.

In 2000, we may have both been willing to compromise and sacrifice for each other, but it was Kristin who actually did it. It's too cliché to say hers was an act I would never forget and always appreciate. Sooner or later, I knew I would have an opportunity to demonstrate my love and commitment to her.

That opportunity came unexpectedly several years later when her dad's prostate cancer returned with a vengeance. Her selfless actions during our civil war help explain mine when I resigned my active duty commission without hesitation in 2009 so we could be near him.

I traded in every ounce of influence I had to get us home to Minnesota. When that failed, I reached out to General Petraeus for help. His personal note to a fellow general officer ended, "The only remaining step is to have the open requisition validated by your command—a step I hope you can take, as it will help both that program and a great officer and his family."

I had orders for the University of Minnesota ROTC program as an executive officer *within twelve hours*. I had never seen anything move that fast in the army. I swelled with pride and felt a lump in my throat as I called Kristin over to the computer. I watched her eyes scan the e-mail and saw the reality sink in. Then I spoke as if I were opening a surprise anniversary gift. "Honey, I'm taking you home." We shared a long, tearful hug.

☆ ☆ ☆

Each of you boys, in your own way, has come to me and asked why Kristin and I fight the way we do. In each case, there is an assumed question about how it is that two people can fight so passionately and still claim to love one another.

I propose to you that it is virtually impossible to find or maintain a relationship that won't come with fights, and that love and a good marriage is not about avoiding fights—it's about fighting fair and making up.

The same questions have been asked about how we get along when we have such pronounced differences in taste. There's lots of debate on this one in academic circles, but not to me. I would never choose the music your mom listens to, but because I love her, I think of her when I hear a song I know she likes. I've never had a problem liking her music in that context—or your music, for that matter. And I didn't have to stop being me to do it.

Finally, all my adult life, I have struggled with making sure I provided the right kind of balance between family and work. I never did know if I got it right, but I did stick to a guiding principle: working hard is critical to the long-term stability of the family, so do it. But when you're home, be home.

I've learned that more time with family is not always better time with family. Quality, reliability, and engagement are the things you all seemed to appreciate the most.

Me, too.

CHAPTER FIVE

... To seek a temper of the will,
a quality of the imagination, and to exercise
a temperamental predominance of courage
over timidity.

March–September 2011

Going back to work after recovering from surgery was exhilarating for me, but it was a bit problematic for the army. Soldiers with terminal cancer don't go back to work. They are thanked for their service and medically retired. And as a career lieutenant colonel, I stood ready to collect a generous pension, so that option made logical sense. Except to me.

Although senior leaders of the Minnesota National Guard found my desire to work at least as puzzling as inspiring, they agreed to support me by offering me a temporary full-time assignment. The arrangement would harness my energy while ensuring minimum disruption to them if my health failed to meet my optimism.

Temper of the will and a quality of the imagination were now required of both me and the army, because this had never been done before.

My tasks weren't busy-work. They included reviewing the strategic planning and performance improvements processes for the Minnesota National Guard, as well as assuming a leading role in improving our efforts with suicide prevention—a challenge that unfortunately put Minnesota, with its particularly high incidence of soldier suicide, in a national spotlight.

Up.

This was the kind of vital assignment I'd wanted when I first came into the organization, and I threw myself into it so thoroughly that the job was eventually made permanent, and I was promoted to the position of director of strategic communication.

Down.

My health had wavered frequently in the weeks leading into March—usually two or three weeks of feeling great, followed by three days of illness with the knock-down power of the worst flu you ever had.

Either the surgery or the cancer growth was causing bile to back up inside my liver and leech into my body, which led to *sepsis*, a deadly infection I would intimately come to know: thirty to sixty minutes of violent, shaking chills; vomiting; white stool; orange urine; head-to-toe itching and body aches; burning, yellow eyes and skin; and a migraine-like headache.

This form of sepsis carries a 60-percent mortality rate, which always seemed accurate because I truly wondered if I were going to survive the night each time it happened—at least thirty times in two years.

Up.

To fix the sepsis problem, radiologists inserted a catheter through my ribs, across my liver, and straight down through the bile duct (a Pixy-Stix-size tube that connects the liver to the body). One end of the catheter drains into my intestine; the other end is connected to a drainage bag that hangs from the space between my ribs. In essence, they installed a drain, so the liver would never again back up like a clogged sink.

Down.

Starting in March, each successive CT scan showed the cancer was still growing, which indicated a failing Gleevec chemo response. Still, Gleevec is the most promising drug on the market for GIST patients, so we all anxiously and patiently waited from March until August before concluding that it had failed.

The doctors followed the standard protocol of doubling the dose.

Up and down.

In August, after four months without a major bout of sepsis, the doctors decided to remove the catheter in my liver in the hopes my damaged bile duct had healed.

Also, a CT scan showed the double dose of Gleevec was working extremely well, which was a welcome gift on the one-year "cancerversary" of my diagnosis.

But in September, just a few weeks later, I experienced a bout of sepsis serious enough to put me in the hospital. The scar tissue on the bile duct was still blocking the flow of bile, so the catheter had to go back into my liver. (And hasn't come out since.)

Worse, Buford started acting up; an abscess the size of a silver dollar formed right on the incision line and deep in the abdominal muscle, which affected everything I did. I could still get around and push through a day of work, but the pain was almost unbearable for a week until the antibiotics kicked in.

Somebody stop the ride. I want to get off.

Amidst all the ups, downs, and uncertainties of this six-month period in 2011, "you should write a book" became a common refrain from those who followed my online CaringBridge journal.

I rejected the idea of writing a formal memoir, but the constant suggestion did convince me there might be some merit in sorting through twenty-two years of journal entries to organize my life experience for you boys.

★ ★ ★

When Samuel Ullman wrote the refrain in this chapter's title some forty years prior to MacArthur's speech, he was not speaking of leadership, patriotism, or duty. He was speaking of *youth*, which is also the title of his poem, excerpted here:

Whether sixty or sixteen, there is in every human being's heart the lure of wonder, the unfailing child-like appetite of what's next, and the joy of the game of living.

In the center of your heart and my heart there is a wireless station; so long as it receives messages of beauty, hope, cheer, courage and power from men and from the infinite, so long are you young.

When the [sails] are down, and your spirit is covered with snows of cynicism and the ice of pessimism, then you are grown old, even at twenty, but as long as your [sails] are up, to catch the waves of optimism, there is hope you may die young at eighty.

But if you're going to die young when you're old, you must first *be* young when you are young. And I was young.

I spent my last semester in college at Nicollet Public School as a student teacher for seventh through twelfth grades. To say I embraced it with a temperamental idealism would be an understatement. As a soon-to-be army lieutenant, I saw this as a real-world opportunity to practice what I had learned about leadership and management—and with *teenagers*, no less.

Things went reasonably well for most of the semester. Most of the kids seemed entertained by their temporary new monkey (me), and I really felt as if I were connecting. I taught with fire and passion. But one of the teachers warned my style was not sustainable.

"You'll burn out," she said. This comment came as no surprise to me, because her teaching style was about as interesting as wet paint.

Two weeks from graduation, all hell broke loose. I had just finished teaching a section on the American Civil War in my tenth-grade history class. I posed a question for the class: "The slaves are all free, so now what?"

One boy in the front row, a routine rabble-rouser, blurted out, "Kill the niggers." The room froze, and I heard audible gasps from other students.

Without yelling, I ordered him with a wave of my finger, "You get the hell out of my classroom. Go down to the principal's office, and tell him what you said to get kicked out of my class."

Just then, another voice arose from the back of the room. "I don't see what he said was so wrong." It was a buddy who decided to support his embattled friend.

"Go on—go join your buddy, big mouth," I told him.

The principal, ironically nicknamed "Whitey," told me to determine a punishment with his full support. After consulting with my host teacher, Brad Koenig, I settled on in-school suspension, which would require the sacrifice of a Saturday under my supervision.

Two days later, I was called to the main office and told the district superintendent, Mr. John Booth, wanted to see me. His office was housed in our school, but I had never met the man.

As I approached his door, I noticed a woman I did not recognize sitting in front of his desk. Her face said "anxious" with a bullhorn. As I entered the room, I saw the "wet paint" teacher standing next to the suspended boys, both of whom looked awfully confident.

"Come over here behind my desk by me, Mr. Weber," Booth said calmly and with a forced smile.

I smelled an ambush. And I took note that Whitey was out of town.

"Mr. Weber," Booth said warmly, "I've brought you in here to discuss what happened earlier this week in your class with these boys." He introduced the anxious woman as one of the mothers, then explained that he invited Mrs. Wet Paint to help provide perspective.

His recap of events was notable in two ways: short on the details of the boys' behavior and heavy handed regarding my use of the word *hell*. He compared our behaviors as if they were cut from the same cloth, and then suggested I reconsider the suspensions.

"I don't see how my behavior has anything to do with what these boys did," I said, sounding desperate and pathetic.

"Well," Booth replied, "this isn't something we need the boys in here to discuss." He dismissed them with a wave of his hand and a fatherly tone, "You two head on back to class now. Your suspensions are revoked."

My heart raced. I slowly moved from behind the desk. After a few moments of silence, I muttered, "I don't . . . um . . . I don't understand what just happened here."

Mrs. Wet Paint spoke first with some backhanded comment about my teaching style, which Booth repeated like a parrot.

I glared at her, "What does *my teaching style* have to do with what those boys did?" But it was plain enough that I was outnumbered and outgunned, so I didn't press the matter.

I left that office in a daze. I went to discuss with Koenig what had happened, but the day was almost over, and it was Friday.

Sadness and intimidation quickly turned to steel resolve—I may have been a student teacher, but something stunk here, and I was *not* going to take it lying down.

I undertook my own investigation that weekend and was shocked at what I found. Booth was in a probationary employment status as superintendent; he had a history of alcohol and drug abuse that included at least one DWI.

As in most school districts across the country, Booth served at the pleasure of the school board. And that anxious mother I met in Booth's office was *president* of the school board.

Del Vulcan was a parent with three kids enrolled in Nicollet. He was also a lieutenant colonel in the army, my senior mentor, and head of the ROTC department at Minnesota State University. When he confirmed what I had learned, my decision about what to do next was clear. I would seek a private meeting with Booth man to man and propose a solution that would punish me but also reinstate the boys' suspensions. *The plan briefed well.*

I confidently strolled into the school on Monday morning, wearing my truth and reason like a suit of armor. I sought nothing for myself; surely Booth would see virtue in that.

I spoke with Booth in the most respectful tone I could muster as I asked him to reconsider his judgment about the matter. When I finished, he leaned back in his chair, chuckled, and mocked my presence in his office. In that moment, Booth looked like the caricature of a crooked villain in a James Bond movie.

He stood up and moved to a seat adjacent to me and explained in a patronizing tone, "Mr. Weber, I'll tell you what you're going to do. You're going to go back to your class, and you're going to finish out your last few weeks of student teaching experience here at Nicollet."

So it comes to this, then, I thought.

I braced myself in my chair and spoke with conviction. "I need to be more clear," I said. "I'm not going back into that classroom until you tell those boys what they did was wrong." Then I calmly, but directly, laid out each of the facts: "I know you're on probation as the superintendent here, and I know what influential position that mother holds on the school board."

The look on his speechless face wasn't much different from Billy Bean's years ago.

As emboldened as I felt, I practically lowered my head as I pleaded with him, "Look, the door is closed, and it's just you and me here. Why won't you see that this is the right thing to do? Punish me, hold me accountable for my behavior, but tell those boys what they did was wrong." I thought for certain that humility would grip him, but instead he was incensed.

The hair on my neck stood on end as he glared at me and raised his voice, "*Don't . . . you . . . dare* tell me how to run this school, young man. You are speaking to the superintendent of this school *district*! Now you get your things together and get back to your class *now*!"

"I will not, sir," I replied calmly. "You have stripped me of my authority and sent a clear message to those students, as well as to other teachers, about who runs the show around here. I cannot return until those kids know otherwise." Booth stood up, reached behind me, opened the door, and raised his voice again, "I've had enough of this—now you get the hell out of my office, or you're done here."

I stood up, looked him straight in the face, and calmly said, "Mr. Booth, you are a coward."

Holy shit. I think I physically saw the top of his head come unglued from his skull. "That's it, mister! You—are—fired! You get your shit, and you get out of this school right *now*!"

I was shaken to the core. *How could I be so right and end up so wrong?*

Koenig's twelfth-grade class was in session when I entered the room. His look told me he could read my face. "What's wrong?" he said.

That question unlocked my emotions, and my eyes filled with tears. "It's over," I said. "He fired me."

The bell rang, and those students poured into that hallway like gossips on a mission from God. Hearing about the firing turned an already juicy story into an instant legend, and they didn't even have the details yet. Many of my students—mostly my seventh graders—approached me at the doorway to Koenig's classroom with tears in their eyes, asking if it were true.

A few weeks later, the school board met, and the sight was

unprecedented. I had been asked to come and speak, because a host of parents wanted to hear from me. Koenig later remarked he'd never seen anything like it in twenty-five years of teaching. "Seeing that many angry parents was impressive enough, but seeing equally angry students aligned with their parents was priceless."

Booth opened with an announcement, "Now I want to be clear here that this meeting is not going to be about Mr. Weber. We have important school business to tend to here." (Koenig later remarked, "What the hell did he think all those parents were there to discuss? The school's fuel bill?")

The standing ovation and vote of confidence I received from parents and students that night was intoxicating, but it didn't relieve me of feeling like a failure for my temperamental approach.

Of course, there was something universally noble about standing up to Booth, but he never did rebuke those boys. And had this been a real job, I'm not so sure nobility would have counted for much in the unemployment line. There was plenty of room in which to feel proud, but also to seek better balance.

✷ ✷ ✷

Tempered wills and temperamental tendencies aren't just for bosses. It can be just as difficult to find courage when dealing with respected peers and subordinates.

In late June 1996, the Khobar Towers complex in Saudi Arabia was bombed. Nineteen US airmen were killed, and more than 370 personnel were wounded. The complex, which consisted of a few dozen tightly packed, eight-story condos, was home to about four thousand US soldiers and airmen stationed in the country.

After the bombing, the Department of Defense made a decision to repatriate all US family members back to the states and move all US service members into a more defendable location. An order was drafted for fifty MP soldiers and one MP officer to help carry out the mission.

The excitement in the Triple Nickel was conspicuous when that order arrived at Fort Lee. Real-world missions like this were rare in the '90s, and the size and scope of the task were twice what any platoon leader would normally lead. These facts made it a dream assignment, and the task fell to me.

Our expectations were high—and they were shattered almost immediately upon arrival in Saudi Arabia, where we were assigned to OPM-SANG, a rank-heavy US Army command that would serve as our "parents" during the deployment.[5]

My fifty-man team was split into four groups and scattered throughout a country the size of the western United States. The work our soldiers received was akin to mall security and would ultimately have nothing to do with security for US families; fifty German shepherds would have served the same purpose.

Ninety percent of the personnel in OPM-SANG were majors and lieutenant colonels, a stark contrast in age, experience, and expectations compared with my enlisted soldiers. This environment made conditions ripe for conflict, which was ignited at the top.

Several of our young soldiers were verbally reprimanded by senior officers for wearing shorts and flip-flops to the community pool. Command policy required all soldiers to respect local customs and wear head-to-toe clothing while walking to and from the pool, because local Saudis worked in the compound. The policy and the reprimand were appropriate, except for one thing: senior officers routinely violated the policy themselves.

The idea of taking up this issue with a general officer twenty-five years senior in experience and rank wore hard on me in light of the still-fresh experience at Nicollet with Mr. Booth, but I felt the same conviction to do the right thing.

Just don't call the man a coward, and we'll be okay.

---

5.   Office of the Program Manager–Saudi Arabian National Guard (OPM-SANG) is a thirty-plus-year-old US Army organization responsible for training and advising the roughly one hundred thousand soldiers in the Saudi National Guard, a domestic security force for the kingdom that is *separate* from the Saudi armed forces.

I enlisted the support of a lieutenant colonel sixteen years senior to me to provide "flank support" and then personally took up the case with the general.

When I met with Brigadier General Larry Smith, we engaged in pleasant small talk, then he invited me to speak my mind.

"Sir, I need your help," I began. "My soldiers violated the uniform policy, and I need to fix that—I can take care of that. I'd like to ask *your* help in getting the senior officers to help set the example."

Smith leaned back in his chair and literally spoke down the brim of his nose at me. His condescending tone was even more pronounced than Mr. Booth's had been.

"Now you listen up, *Lieutenant* Weber," he said softly. "We're not going to get into that kind of talk and comparison around here. This issue doesn't belong at my level." (Actually, it did.) "You just take care of your platoon of soldiers. They're doing a fine job, and you just need to make sure they keep that up." Without skipping a beat, he shifted to a more upbeat tone and choice of subject, "Aren't these facilities just grand? Now, how's your family doing?"

What grace. What skill. *What slime.*

I glanced over at my flank for support, but the colonel stood there like a sheep. He didn't even try.[6]

It was bad enough getting shot down by someone like Smith. It was far worse getting shot down by a respected subordinate in the incident that followed.

Despite the total letdown in expectations with the Saudi mission, I decided to focus on the one thing that meant the most in any case—the welfare of our soldiers and their families.

I talked one on one with soldiers and junior leaders about their work conditions and off-duty likes and dislikes, and I wrote a news-

---

6. Four years later, I saw General Smith's face on the cover of *The Army Times* for sexual harassment and a forced retirement from the army. It felt good knowing that he ended up in the unemployment line with Mr. Booth.

letter to families back home describing our living arrangements and the hundreds of dollars in extra income we were making.

Everyone liked the attention and the involvement, except Sergeant First Class Avery James. He was my new platoon sergeant, and he was actually the kind of NCO I had dreamed of getting nearly three years prior. But with the newsletter, he thought I was too involved and shared too much information.

"It's a private matter," he insisted, regarding the money details. "Some soldiers don't want their spouses knowing about the extra income so close to the holidays." And he had come from the school of thought that soldier welfare was the sole domain of the NCO.

More than anything, however, he resented things I had no control over. We had no vehicles or equipment to maintain, little or no time for individual training or weapons marksmanship, no logistical supplies to coordinate, and soldiers who were farmed out all over the country.

These conditions relieved James of roughly 90 percent of his job as an NCO, a condition that was accentuated by the fact that there was a 50-to-1 ratio of officers to NCOs. I shared his frustration, but there was nothing I could do about it, and he knew it.

My dustup and subsequent failure with General Smith only further incensed James. His resentment for our environment spread to a resentment toward me, and on one occasion, he lashed out at me in front of a few soldiers. Without even thinking, I ordered him outside, acknowledged his frustration about the circumstances, and then laid into him.

"What is it exactly that you think we're supposed to do here, mutiny?" I asked him. "Am I supposed to place my rank on the table and offer a threat of resignation because of all this?"

As much as we disliked the mission, we really had nothing to complain about. We were receiving combat and hazardous duty pay for conditions that were anything *but* hazardous. Ours was a collective mismanagement of expectations, and I told him he needed to help our soldiers extinguish their fires of discontent, not throw fuel on them.

James's insubordination in front of soldiers is a cardinal sin in the army. I thought about his exceptional performance to date as the next thought made it to my lips: "I can handle disagreements in private, but if that kind of public insubordination ever happens again, I will do all in my power to have you redeployed to the states on the very first plane out of the country."

Personally, I still wonder what he thought of me in that moment, but professionally, the only thing I cared about was him changing his crappy attitude. To his credit, he did just that.

When you're in charge, everyone knows how to do things better than you are doing them. That was no exception with Second Lieutenant Mike Burns. Our deployment called for only one officer, but Burns was sent anyway, so his presence was already redundant and unwelcome from day one.

Still wet behind the ears in the army, let alone as an officer, Burns had a very immature professional attitude.

"You're just not forceful enough with these jokers," he'd say with a casual wave of his hand. He had clever retorts about working with senior officers that revealed a warped understanding of the profession.

"Schmoozing isn't my style," he'd say. "I speak only when spoken to." He found staff meetings to be tedious, which they are, but he seemed to have missed the fact that they came with the territory.

Burns's loose attitude came to him honestly, as he worked mostly at night and out of sight of senior officers. But I was just as direct with him when he criticized me in front of our soldiers for the same issues James did.

I held a razor-thin line of superiority over Burns, so imagination, unconscious as it was on my part, had to be the tactic of choice. I told him I was assigning him new duties. He would join me in the headquarters on the day shift for a little firsthand senior officer experience and professional perspective.

I imagined he would be disappointed, but I had no idea it would make him as angry as it did. He tried reasoning with me and even apologized for offending me, but I had no intention of letting the matter go. "No . . . it's about time you had the opportunity to show me how to do it right."

He recoiled hard. "I don't need to experience it to know how it should be done. When you're right, you're right, and that's all you need."

I thought about my experience with Booth as well as the recent run-in with Smith, and I replied, "I somehow missed the lesson that teaches that you can still get your way when folks who outrank you don't listen or don't care what you think."

"You're not in charge of shit!" he yelled. "You're not the commander!" His quick call back to the states was short. He showed up the next morning for his appointed duties and developed (I'd like to think) a new appreciation for the context of tempered wills and temperamental tendencies.

✮ ✮ ✮

Nearly two years after my adventures in Saudi Arabia, I was assigned to a job that seemed to punctuate the importance of risking failure and missteps in the practice of MacArthur's proposal. In fact, "temper of the will" would become as much about softening as hardening—for both the subordinate and the superior.

On the week of my promotion to the rank of captain in 1998, my boss told me the brigade commander, Colonel John Della Jacono ("DJ," for short), wanted me to compete for assignment as his senior logistics officer (brigade S4). Far from being flattered, I was terrified. The job was rated for a major, not a captain (certainly not a newly minted captain). And I was a military policeman, not a logistics officer.

Responsibilities included logistical oversight of five battalions totaling about 800 instructors and 1,800 soldiers, a $1.2-million annual budget, and $4.5 million in contractual obligations for weapons ranges and dining facilities.

The duties were intimidating enough, but added to the equation was the fact that Fort McClellan would permanently close in fifteen months. This meant the new brigade S4 would also have to account for everything in the vast organization—thousands and thousands of pieces of furniture, equipment, and property—then turn it in or move it to the new brigade's home at Fort Leonard Wood, Missouri. In other words—*double the normal workload.* No thanks!

But before I knew it, I was sitting in front of DJ for an interview. He was cordial, but direct. "So, tell me why I should select you to be my S4," he asked.

"Ah, sir, I think there's been a mistake," I replied. "I didn't express any interest in being the S4, and honestly I don't think I'm qualified in experience or rank." I wasn't trying to be modest. I simply knew my limits. I also knew rank and authority *mattered*; most of the officers I would have to work with would be majors and lieutenant colonels with *years* of experience.

DJ shifted topics, and we spent most of our time focused on things that had nothing to do with logistics. I left his office confident he would pick the senior captain or one of the two majors who had applied for the job, one of whom was a career logistician.

About a week after that interview, I was told my new assignment to the brigade staff was effective immediately. DJ later explained that he knew my rank and experience would offer some unique challenges, but he liked my character and personality. He said he saw an officer who knew how to work hard and wasn't afraid to be bold, and he thought that was going to matter more than anything else with the challenges ahead.

I was furious. I thought DJ's judgment was shortsighted foolishness. I already felt that I was in over my head with my master's program in history at Jacksonville State University. Kristin and I had just been forced to leave our rented home and were in the process of moving onto the base. And changing to a new job beyond my grade and experience would be like sending me into a boxing ring with one arm tied behind my back. *Would it be my fault if I couldn't get the work done to standard?*

As it turned out, the attributes DJ spoke about did make up for my lack of rank and experience in a thousand little ways over the next fifteen months. I was even asked to perform tasks outside my duties. When DJ saw my presentations and written products, he signed me up to prepare briefings for the installation commanding general and asked me to write his speech for the deactivation ceremony of the brigade.

On the one hand, it felt great being able to contribute in such unique ways. On the other hand, I knew I was doing extra work because others weren't willing or able to do theirs, and that really pissed me off—just as it had when I was a kid I and was "rewarded" with most of the household cleaning chores because I was "so good at it."

Not everything went well in my assignment. Having a can-do attitude and fresh perspective was appealing, but with no rank or formal training and experience, I was like a kid trying to wear his dad's suit. This put me at a great disadvantage when there were differences of opinion about big decisions. It wasn't uncommon to get looks from people that screamed, "Who the hell do you think you are, *captain?*"—even from DJ, who loved it when I did bold things for him, but scoffed if I did them on my own.

One event in particular underscored this paradox.

The officer taking DJ's place at Fort Leonard Wood was Rod Johnson, an easygoing and mild-mannered personality who had recently been promoted to colonel. (Eight years later, he would become the provost marshal general of the army.) Johnson was a stark contrast to DJ, who was a fiery, temperamental combat veteran of the 82nd Airborne Division.

During one of our planning meetings at Fort Leonard Wood, Johnson asked if we had any money that we could spare for his fledgling command. He had been given a shoestring budget, and asked if we could spare about $4,000, which was like asking for pocket change, considering the cost of the move. But out of respect for my boss, I didn't reveal we had $85,000 left over in the budget that we were not going to use at Fort McClellan.

When I returned to Alabama and raised the issue with DJ, his answer was an immediate and emphatic, "No!" He was downright dismissive. "You know what they're spending their money on there? Furniture. *Brand-new furniture*, for God's sake!" he fumed. He thought such money should be spent on soldier equipment or not at all. As far as he was concerned, senior officers could sit at a card table.

DJ wasn't alone in his assessment, but the "new furniture" issue was a real problem for Johnson. The army had no intention of spending $10,000 to move beat-up, worn-out, 1970s-vintage, steel desks and chairs from Alabama to Missouri. And the bottom line was that Johnson's staff needed desks and chairs to do their job.

I pleaded with DJ, "Sir, this is money we don't need, and it's a pretty insignificant sum of money in the grand scheme of things." The conversation lasted a good fifteen minutes, and he started to get upset, so I let it drop. Then I paid a visit to the officer who managed everyone's money at Fort McClellan to see if I could find another way to meet the request.

"Why don't you just send the money from your account?" the officer said with a puzzled look on his face. "The transfer is legal, and the money is available in excess. Why are you coming to me to do it for you?" Of course, I wasn't going to tell him that DJ didn't want to.

I weighed all the information I had in hand, banked on my

reputation with DJ as a standup officer (which he'd said he liked when he hired me), and then conducted the money transfer.

A week later DJ called me to his office, confirmed my actions, and then leveled the most devastating ass-chewing I have ever received in my life—then or since. "*You* are a *captain*! I am a *colonel*! What is it that you don't understand about that, Weber?" And that was the politest part of the exchange.

My explanations didn't seem to matter at all. He wasn't more than four inches from my face, and there is no doubt everyone in the surrounding offices heard it. I saw his objection coming, but I did not anticipate the degree of outrage—not after all we had done together.

Still, as shortsighted as DJ's order may have been, telling me not to transfer the money was lawful, which made me dead wrong to disobey. I walked out of his office dizzy and a little numb and went to an abandoned classroom down the hall to try and collect myself.

The incident made me question everything I thought I knew about leading and managing in tough environments. My annual evaluation was due in two weeks, and I concluded I had horribly misjudged a whole host of professional issues.

I didn't think my career was over (army officers can be melo-dramatic about what actually ends a career), but I wondered if this one incident was going to take the shine off a year of back-breaking labor.

When I finally sat down for my evaluation, DJ revealed an example of professionalism I have carried with me ever since. He set aside his personal hang-ups and gave me the most impressive evaluation I had ever seen. A week later, he pinned a Meritorious Service Medal on my chest, an award normally reserved for his commanders.

A few days later at a golf outing over a couple of beers, DJ shared a moment of candor that still warms my heart today. He nearly gushed, telling me how proud he was of the work I had done, and that my efforts over the previous year had ultimately proved him right in selecting me for the job. Clearly, he'd had doubts.

Ten years later, I experienced the same sort of rub with a boss in the Pentagon. Shortly after our assignment was complete, we shared a similar moment, which speaks volumes about the "cuts both ways" nature of being bold, courageous, and imaginative:

> *You were a pain, but I'd rather have had you pushing programs than anyone else. You have a certain verve that can't be suppressed. Once you launch there is very little a boss can do to adjust your trajectory, but you always seem to find the objective and accomplish the mission. It was just a little unsettling getting used to your unusual creativity, drive, and determination. I came to appreciate you though. We wish you were with us now... We could really use some of that old Weber magic that made the impossible happen.*

Tempered wills, imagination, and temperamental tendencies clearly require ruffling feathers and tipping over apple carts to spur the team to solutions.

✳ ✳ ✳

How much effort is enough effort? How far is too far? How hard, how soft, how unpredictable or excitable? How much imagination? Again, I can only offer observations and a few illustrations like the ones above, not clear-cut answers.

When I reflect on the word temper, *I think balance, moderation, and compromise—softening and hardening, not unyielding or impenetrable. There is a point, after all, when your tempered will becomes zealotry or a suicide pact, and your intemperance toward timidity becomes reckless. Through trials and countless errors, I've learned that being reasonable and levelheaded carries great utility in work, politics, religion, money, and love.*

It is striking to me that despite the timeless virtue of finding common ground and practical solutions, too many people fear that such thinking will make them appear weak or lacking in conviction. All I can tell you is that this has not been my experience at all. In fact, it's not even really reflective of the American experience as a whole.

I propose to you that you'll find answers to your questions by taking just one step beyond what others tell you that you shouldn't. Be curious and ask just one more question. Be persistent and insist on just one more consideration. Speak out. At least try.

Be as prepared as Ullman would be (and MacArthur likely would not) *to sit down before every fact as a little child, to give up every preconceived notion, and to follow humbly wherever and to whatever abysses nature leads.*[7] *And when—not if—failure comes, you'll be much stronger and wiser for it.*

---

7.   Adapted from T. H. Huxley, 1860.

CHAPTER SIX

... To be modest (humble) so that you will
appreciate the open mind of true wisdom, and
the meekness (gentleness) of true strength.

October–December 2011

With the arrival of fall and the cold Minnesota weather, the cancer
once again took on the characteristics of hibernating flies—down,
but not out.

Things finally seemed stable, but the calm didn't even last a
month. The silver-dollar-size abscess that had developed on Buford
in September returned just a few weeks later, the antibiotics stopped
working, and the pain was worse. I had rarely rated pain over five
on a scale of ten, so my doctors took notice when I rated Buford
a nine.

My medical team was baffled. One doctor cut into the abscess
with a scalpel and even tried draining it with a syringe, but he got
nothing but blood. "This is incredible," he said. "I've never seen

anything like it. I expected fluid to come gushing out, by the looks of this thing." A scan didn't show them anything either, and I had no other symptoms of infection. If I could tolerate the pain, they wanted me to simply observe and see what happened as my body attempted to resolve it.

That was Thursday afternoon.

By 3:30 a.m. Saturday, I'd had enough. Armed with a small Swiss Army knife and believing I could hardly do worse than the ER at this point, I cut into Buford, deep and wide.

Once.

Then twice.

That abscess burst open like a scene from *Alien*. I don't know where the hell all that fluid had been hiding two days earlier, but I found it deep, past the muscular wall. I could fit my index finger in that hole all the way past the first knuckle.[8]

Until then, we were all convinced Buford's recurrent abscesses were the result of surgical stitches that had not dissolved. But as I stood over a sink filled with stinky, thick, yellow-and-white goo, I smelled an odor that remained sharp in my memory from the year prior. Bile.

My surgeon, Dr. Tim Sielaff, was politely dismissive about my theory. "It can't be bile . . . that would be crazy . . . *craaazy*." A fistula (hole in the intestine) near the liver would have revealed itself long before now. Wouldn't it?

Sielaff knew what I did not: intestinal fistulas following a Whipple procedure are incredibly complicated messes that can persist for years if they don't heal in the first several months after surgery. He didn't *want* it to be a fistula.

The abscess scene above played out four more times over the next three months. My flesh would always heal; the intestinal tissue would not; the bile would collect in the muscular wall and start digesting

---

8.   The medically curious and strong of stomach may see photos section at www. caringbridge.org/visit/markmweber.

the newly healed flesh; and within a few days of searing and unbearable pain, it would burst.

Self-surgery and first-person post-op care became freakishly routine. Although my actions were arguably overly aggressive, I wasn't exactly a medical novice by now. After all, I had nursed an open wound ten times this size, and I knew how to pack wounds as well. My doctors and nurses couldn't condone what I had done, but telling me they wished all their patients were as knowledgeable and persistent was all the affirmation I needed.

Despite our collective understanding, my doctors shared our frustration as each of the experiments failed.

We all took the continued ups and downs in stride—Kristin, me, you boys, my colleagues at work. That's when life threw us another knuckleball. Kristin's mother was diagnosed with brain cancer. (After three invasive surgeries, the cancer is still active.) Prior to that point, we heard a frequent refrain from well-wishers: "God only gives you what you can handle."

Until now.

✳ ✳ ✳

"The open mind of true wisdom" is something I didn't begin to appreciate until college. But even as a kid, there was one subject that always itched but was never really scratched to my satisfaction—*my religion*.

For twelve years—*from age five to eighteen*—I attended a Catholic school, weekly Mass, and Sunday School. Questions weren't discouraged, but they didn't need to be. God's wrath and the burning fires of hell were the undercurrents of the instruction, which hardly encouraged *open* discussion.

None of my other school subjects came with such mystery or incomprehensible consequences for being wrong.

Seeing Jesus up on that cross and reading about his suffering made the entire story—from the virgin birth to his resurrection

from the dead—plenty compelling. Christianity wasn't that difficult to grasp as a young boy:

"*Yes, Jesus loves me, 'cause the Bible tells me so,*" went the song.

"*Jesus died for all of mankind, so that all sin could be forgiven,*"
went the refrain.

"*The price for salvation and everlasting life has been paid for on
the cross. This is the redemptive power of Christ!* (And no other religion has it, by the way.)"

It was easy to believe in such agreeable ideas. With respect and
without mockery, my innocent young mind also had no trouble at
all believing in Santa Claus, the Tooth Fairy, and the Easter Bunny.

I was taught that if I believed strongly enough and prayed hard
enough, God would answer my prayers.

Sometimes this concept was explained as metaphor: *Prayer and
reflection was but one task, and God's answer was the inspiration we
needed to do the rest of the work ourselves.*

Far more often, however, the concept was explained literally: *Prayer and request was our work, and God's answer was direct
intervention.* There *were* words about the importance of personal
responsibility, but those words were greatly overshadowed by the
emphasis on *God's* actions.

The idea of prayer-as-work naturally carried more appeal.
"Dear God, just for this big game, help me keep the puck out of
the net." And the concept cut both ways. If I hurt myself, my mom
half-jokingly said, "See, God is punishing you." And I learned that,
when praying, it was critical to add humble caveats: "If it's your
divine plan or will to do so."

Sometimes it worked. Improbably, our hockey team won the
playoff game. Grandma Garofalo survived her stroke. Much more
often, it did not work. We lost the championship game. Grandma
Weber died after her heart attack. The difference between the two
was explained as a "mystery of faith."

These contradictions spread to numerous other parts of my

religious understanding in much more meaningful ways.

At each Sunday service, we heard stories about a vengeful and egotistical God—one who flooded the earth and killed all but one family of mankind, and later loved *one special* group of humans so much that he personally aided them in *brutally* crushing their enemies on earth.

In the next story, from the same Sunday service, we learned about a God who *unconditionally* loved *all* mankind so much that he sent his son to die *for all of us*.

Having sex outside of marriage was considered sinful and evil. I got that. But even thinking about it was considered the same thing, and I resented the idea that I should feel perverted or shameful for experiencing a biological drive in puberty that was as powerful as hunger.

Suicide bought a ticket straight to the eternal fires of hell, and being a homosexual seemed to carry the same weight as violating one of the Ten Commandments.

Ultimately, if I didn't believe getting into heaven was for Christians alone, I would be welcome to join non-Christians in "not being saved"—which of course meant *going to hell*.

All sorts of translations and explanations—from different priests and religious teachers on the same topics—were offered to help answer my cautious questions, but nothing satisfied me. A sixteen-year-old knows *conditions and mind-spinning contradictions* when he hears them.

This was the instruction, and it was often presented in a very matter-of-fact, nonnegotiable way. I learned to keep my mouth shut and abide by the guidance: "Contradictions and unanswered prayers are the mystery of God's will and work on earth. The strength of your belief in this mystery is a reflection of the strength of your faith."

When it came to prayer, I struggled with the Gregorian chants we had to recite at school and at church, and I found it frustrating talking with people who could only speak in Bible passages. So I distinctly remember the day I received "permission" to do it my way. I heard a reading from the Bible that advised against long, redundant prayers. Praying was meant to be done in private, not out in public to impress others with how well you thought you knew or loved God.[9] I began to speak with God as if he were my dad—deferential, but entitled.

My recollection of these formative religious years is arguably incomplete, unfair, and superficial, but that *is* what happens when such a complex subject is introduced to a child.

None of this produced any doubt about my hope and faith in God. What I did begin to doubt was our collective ability to actually hear—or perhaps *listen* to—what God was saying to us.

I entered adulthood with the understanding that I could have an open mind about faith and religion as long as I stayed within established boundaries.

★ ★ ★

When I deployed to Saudi Arabia at age twenty-six, it was as if someone rolled a grenade into my storehouse of knowledge and understanding about everything in life.

The landscape is 830,000 square miles of stupefying desert, with temperatures routinely over 115 degrees. No rain, rivers, or lakes. Civilization didn't seem to "fit" the landscape at all, an anomaly that became more pronounced as I encountered the culture.

Women not only had no rights, they had to cover themselves from head to toe at all times in public. Forget the right to vote; they didn't even have the right to drive a vehicle.

Most of the nation's labor (and its army) consisted of "third-country nationals" who were little more than slave labor and apparently content to be so.

---

9.   I later came to learn the Bible quote was Matthew 6: 5–8.

Religion and the law were one, and the king employed a workforce known as the Mutawwa ("moo-'tah-wah") to enforce every aspect of the religious rules. (I once met a man whose only job was to cut out or blacken any exposed flesh in the photos on magazine covers in the grocery store.)

The concept of punishment was redefined for me when I visited "Chop-Chop Square," the Western term used to describe the massive public square where limbs and, on rare occasion, heads were severed from criminals' bodies.

Surrounding the square was the largest *suq* ("sook"), or open-air market, in Riyadh. *Hey honey, let's take in a public beheading and then get our shopping done while we're there.*

My soldiers viewed this environment with skepticism and distrust. "Fuck this madness, man. These people are crazy. I'm staying in the compound."

But I couldn't. Like an amateur anthropologist, I viewed all of it with wide-eyed and cautious interest. I spent a few nights a week engaging the shopkeepers in the Chop-Chop suq.

Two shopkeepers stood out from the rest. One was Shamsi Obaidi, an unmarried Indian, age twenty-one, with no family. The other was Ahmed Shafik, a married Egyptian, age thirty-one, with one child.

What started as casual experiments in hard bargaining over occasional purchases quickly turned to tea, sweets, and spirited-but-whispered discussions about all manner of topics. In a country where distrust and anxiety are default emotions and a misstep can result in a closed shop and jail time, a visit from an interested and apparently trustworthy American was a welcome respite.

Shamsi came from a wealthy family in India and graduated early from college. His father had big plans for him in Europe but bought a small storefront in Riyadh, where it was easier and less costly to experiment with a business. He left Shamsi to run and manage it all on his own. Shamsi hated it. In India, he had social circles that matched his age and energy; in Saudi Arabia, he was a virtual prisoner. He sat in that shop every day for ten hours, and no one ever took any interest in him outside of business.

If being with Shamsi was like watching a movie, being with Ahmed was like being *in* the movie. Married with a newborn daughter, he was clearly more mature and worldly wise.

Conversations with Ahmed were about the same kinds of things I was experiencing in life—courtship, fatherhood, work, world views. But of all these, our discussions about religion were the most riveting. Our conversations turned my military deployment into an intercultural sabbatical for religious study.

One of our most memorable discussions revolved around the matter of judgment in the afterlife. "The angels, one on the left shoulder and one on the right," he said in his broken English, "they sit in judgment with the book of your life works in the pages. If the scale go one way, you go to the heaven. If the scale go the other way, then the serpent, he come from the ground, and he take you to the hell."

"You really believe that?" I asked. He smiled, took a sip of his tea, and replied in a nonverbal way that he was aware of my disbelief. Then he spoke up, "You believe that the Jesus was born without a father and he die and rise from the dead. How is it that *my* story is so hard to believe?"

I pressed him on the matter of the afterlife. "So, I am an infidel . . ." I started with a big smile. He burst out with nervous laughter. "What will happen to me?" I continued. He stopped laughing and rocked his head from side to side, as if unsure about how to answer, while he sipped his tea.

"Come on, tell me," I said with a playful smile. We both knew how he would answer. Then he looked at me without smiling and said, "I am sorry, my friend, but you will go to the hell."

"Well," I said, "maybe we'll see each other there and both be surprised." That's when he smiled again, and I was thankful to return to less serious topics.

On a later occasion, we addressed the issue of religious values and redemption. "What about the violence and warlike-theme of the Koran," I asked.

"Your Bible is not violent or warlike?" he politely responded.

"Well, we Christians focus on the New Testament, not the Old."

"Really?" he said in a dismissive tone as he looked away. He tilted his head and smiled with a thinly veiled contempt as he rattled off a quick history of Christian behavior since the time of Christ. "The violent message is there for Christians to take as they like, too," he said with confidence.

On the issue of redemption, I pointed out the stark difference between Islam and Christianity, namely that Islam has no redemption. He pressed me, "The Jesus, he die for your sins . . . so you are not judged when you die?" It was clear he was asking me a loaded question, but I wasn't sure how or what.

"No, we *will be* judged," I answered. "But the point is that Jesus died for our sins, so we can all be saved."

"Yes, that is what I said," Ahmed replied. "He die for your sin. You believe this is required for the heaven. Where and when the judgment?" After a few more minutes of confusing discussion, it dawned on me that he was referencing the Christian belief that salvation is about grace and not deeds. If true, what was it, exactly, that we would be judged upon or sent to hell for? *Our words and thoughts?* I had no answer—*for him or for me.*

This wasn't some highhanded twist of logic he was throwing at me. Nor was he arguing for Islam. It was what I said I believed, and it was the best explanation I could give after twenty years of what I thought was thoroughly examined religious conviction. It was the *"God's-unconditional-love-with-conditions-and-stunning-contradictions"* discussion of my youth all over again.

Because most adults I knew were unwilling or unable to have

a discussion that didn't begin and end with a literal and exclusive read of John 14:6—"I am the way, the truth, and the life, no man comes unto the Father except through me"—I was ill equipped for the discussion.

My frustration with Ahmed later turned to acceptance as I saw we were both exercising the same kind of faith with the same kinds of mystery, a conclusion I kept to myself after a family member scoffed at my comparison of Islam to Christianity.

Not once did Ahmed ask me to consider Islam, nor did he ridicule or mock me for being a Christian. He didn't even suggest it. In fact, after several weeks of interaction, he invited me to his home for dinner and treated me like royalty.

Engaging in dozens of exchanges with a Muslim was an amazing cultural experience in and of itself. But I got the bonus plan from the Kingdom of Saudi Arabia.

Every week or so, I brought Ahmed a new VHS movie from the massive library of films in OPM-SANG. On one such visit bringing him the movie *Rob Roy*, I was approached by the infamous Mutawwa. Their bushy beards and long white robes and caps made them stand out amongst the Western-dressed Riyadh populace, but I had never seen one up close until now.

He demanded to see what was in my hand. "*Ish hada, Rob Roy?*" the Mutawwa demanded. I knew enough Arabic to know he was asking, "What is this, *Rob Roy?*"

"That's the name of the movie," I replied in English. I think he understood me, but the answer did not satisfy him. Ahmed suddenly appeared and provided some much-needed translation.

The Mutawwa wanted to know if the video was pornography, which is against the law. He said I was under apprehension and would need to come with him. I knew it was not pornography, so being "taken away" didn't make me as nervous as I now realize it should have made me. Ahmed nervously said he would not leave my side.

The Mutawwa gently took me by the arm and escorted me on

foot across the "Chop-Chop Square" to what looked like a police station.

Minutes after we took a seat in a small room, a well-dressed interrogator came in and spoke to me as if I were trafficking narcotics. I explained that I was a US Army officer, showed him my military identification, and strategically told him I worked with forces that belonged to the Saudi crown prince. That didn't seem to impress him.

After I had been left alone for another thirty minutes, this Saudi Columbo returned again with the same serious attitude. He and "his team" had found a nudity scene in the movie that made the movie pornographic. They decided to let me go, but with a stern warning, "No more American movies *of any kind*."

I wasn't "reborn" in Saudi Arabia, and I wasn't converted. Nor did I suddenly doubt everything about my faith or launch my own personal crusade to discover it. I just realized how stunningly ignorant I was about the *practice* of my faith and life in general. I didn't know anything about the dominant religions of the world, and I didn't have a defensible spiritual philosophy.

This revelation had implications and interests beyond the personal.

As an army officer, I saw how knowledge and understanding of religion and culture was critical to my profession. The number of fanatical Muslims blowing themselves and others up demanded a closer examination.

I started watching Oxford-style debates between Jewish, Christian, and Islamic scholars, and picked up *History of God* by Karen Armstrong (a former Catholic nun). I felt baffled that twelve years of formal Catholic education hadn't exposed me to anything remotely close to such lively and intellectually stimulating discussions. I realized those twelve years were just the introduction.

I learned that wherever a respectful, open-minded religious discussion led, it did not begin with exhortations about exclusive rights to the definition and rights of way to the afterlife.

Most importantly, I learned that Muslims (and followers of other faiths) were not the aliens I had been led to believe they were.

Extremist observers of their practices no more represented their religion than Christian extremists represented mine. They shared common virtues of peace, love, and a *desire* for morality that was every bit as sincere and imperfect as any Christian's I ever knew. In fact, followers of other religions had gone through or were going through their own *violent* internal strife regarding the meaning of *their* religious texts. The struggle is endless.

More to the point, I began to see we're all part of a world where global real estate is shrinking but information and trade are exploding, where conflicting ideologies no longer enjoy the benefit of space or distance. Short of a mass extinction or genocide, if even that, it seemed clear to me that we needed to find ways to coexist in peace.

I didn't need to agree with other religious practices to understand others' reasons for practicing them. Knowing this, it seemed wise to develop a conversation that was deeper than exchanges over who was going to heaven and hell, and instead focus on the virtues we have in common (and there are many).

When I left Saudi Arabia, I was full of pride about how Ahmed and I had carried ourselves. I was full of hope, too. If the two of us could exercise such a respectable discourse over the practice of our faith, couldn't everyone else?

In the several years that followed, I found I had no grand conclusions about what God was or was not. I had questions, and I asked them, but with great caution. Few people seemed willing or able to discuss the topic outside established boundaries, either afraid of or uninterested in tough questions of God or their religion.

The "mystery of faith" flag, it seemed to me, was being thrown *way* too soon in discussions, and the practice was unmistakably grounded in fear.

I began to challenge those who seemed to think they had it all sorted out without asking any tough questions or engaging in thoughtful discussions without judgment—but more so for the sake of challenging and developing myself.

✻ ✻ ✻

Closer to home, and beside the realm and declared virtues of religion, I saw the humility of open-minded wisdom and gentleness of true strength in a most unlikely character. I met Command Sergeant Major Jim Barrett in 1997 at Fort McClellan, Alabama, where we worked side by side—he as the highest and most respected *enlisted* rank in the army, and I the most junior and least respected *officer* rank in the army.

Jim came from a hard scrabble youth immersed in alcohol, drugs, crime, and family turmoil. His parents divorced when he was five, and his forty-one-year-old father drank himself to death when Jim was twelve. His mother remarried, but was divorced again by the time he turned sixteen. Jim dropped out of high school and essentially turned into a trouble-making bum. Had it not been for Paula, his girlfriend at the time (who would become his wife), he would have participated in a robbery that ended in the arrest of his friends.

One year out of school and seeing his life going nowhere fast, Jim met an army recruiter. But the army doesn't take dropouts. Armed with a new sense of purpose and direction for his energies, he shed his old ways and old friends, returned to school, and worked with such fever that he actually graduated on time with his class.

Jim came off as a New Jersey knuckle-dragger, but he was the most competent soldier I'd ever met. And the combination made him intimidating. He was always right, but not in a *"you've always gotta be right, don't you?"* kind of way. He was the first to teach me that doing your best and making it one's business to *be* right wasn't a vice—it was a reflection of competence that was distressing only to the lazy, insecure, or incompetent.

Life was painful for those who wanted to try psychoanalyzing his motives. Me? I latched on to him like a student to a master. And he reciprocated without me even knowing it. Years after my written reprimand for crawling through the Kramers' bedroom window, I found out Jim was my strongest defender.

"I think it's commendable that you didn't just sit back and watch a situation go from bad to worse—you saw a problem and did something about it. Now, in the future don't go climbing through windows, because you might get hit in the head with a bat."

When we weren't watching WWF wrestling with his two boys, Jimmy and Jeffrey, he was providing counsel on how to take care of soldiers. For years, I saw the familiarity he mixed in with the discipline of his boys (and soldiers) did not make him weak or ineffective as a father (or as a leader).

He helped me see nuances in my professional leadership, too. "I don't believe in 'NCO business,'" he would say, referring to work to be performed solely by sergeants. "There are things NCOs focus on, and there are things officers focus on, and that relationship is unique in every partnership. For me, if an officer has to do something an NCO normally does, it means I'm not doing my job, and I can't get mad at the officer for that."

Jim left Alabama, and we didn't see each other again for four years, staying in touch by e-mail and phone while he was in Germany. In those four years, he rose to the most senior position in the MP Corps (regimental command sergeant major), and we ended up stationed together again at Fort Leonard Wood.

As big and important as he had become, our personal and professional relationship picked up right where it left off. It wasn't uncommon for us to spend four hours at night talking in our backyards about leadership or his colorful life growing up in New Jersey.

I came to see that as often as he was right, he was never afraid to be wrong about something or to laugh at himself. He once asked me to come to his house to help him with an Internet connection (in the days when dial-up service was the standard).

"Where's your phone jack?" I asked.

"What the fuck do I need a phone jack for?" he asked in his intentionally crude voice.

We laughed together as I told him, "What, you think the Internet signal just jumps out of the wall into your computer?" He laughed at himself then, and he still does.

Nor was he afraid or shy about seeking advice. Just before we found out about my assignment to Washington, DC, Jim came and asked me about selling his townhome, because he knew that we had sold *our* Virginia home without an agent.

He had bought his home ten years prior for $130,000. He rented it out for seven years, and as a reward for his renters' loyalty, he thought it would be nice to just let them assume the $110,000 he still owed and save the hassle of agent fees and sales negotiations.

I balked. "Look at it this way," I told him. "Assuming the house is still worth only $130,000—and it's probably worth more—you're proposing to *pay your renters* $20,000 to buy this house from you." He owed it to himself to figure out the value of the home and how generous he was really being.

This exchange with Jim told me so much about him as a person. His single mother worked three jobs to raise him and his brother. And he and his wife, Paula, weren't exactly rolling in money at the time. I went home and told Kristin about his incredible personal example. It made me want to be a better person.

About a week later, he called me back. "Holy shit, dude, you're not gonna believe this," he said. "That townhome is worth $180,000—as is!"

I chuckled and reminded him that his earlier decision would have given his renters a $70,000 gift. "Were your renters *that* good?" I asked.

Still, he settled on a $150,000 price tag. The only thing more stunning than his now-$30,000 discount was the fact that his renters turned him down.

"Listen, sergeant major," I told him, "if those fools don't take your offer, I hope you'll offer me the same deal, because even if the house has problems, it's the most generous thing I've ever heard of in my life." We bought it without even looking at it and used every penny of the equity to fix it up.

Four years later when it was time to move again and the housing market was crashing, a real estate agent found out we were trying to sell it on our own and laughed in our face. "There is *no way* you'll sell on your own in this market."

We sold it in less than two weeks.

How?

We followed Jim and Paula's example and sold our home $20,000 below market value. We still made every penny we would have by using an agent, and we "paid it forward." (I also made a point of visiting that agent to return his laugh, in kind.)

That noisy, vulgar Jersey guy taught me how to do that. And in the process, he taught me another lesson in being open-minded.

✷ ✷ ✷

The first time I learned to truly appreciate the value of humility in wisdom regarding politics was in 2003. The army sent me to Georgetown University to spend a year doing nothing but studying the art and science of policy making and politics.

Although soldiers are allowed to express political opinion and even campaign on behalf of candidates, we are restricted from doing so while in uniform, which is harder than it seems. It was far easier to follow the unwritten rule that officers should be politically knowledgeable, but entirely nonpartisan.

I was able to be nonpartisan, but I fell short on being politically knowledgeable. As such, Washington, DC, and Georgetown became the Saudi Arabia of my political awareness.

One of the first things we learned about policy is that there is no ideal solution—*ever*. Formulating policy for a nation of three hundred million citizens is rarely about finding the best or most efficient options and almost always about finding the *least* worst options.

In the end, we all get policies and programs that are more feasible than optimal, more satisfactory than perfect, more tolerable than desirable, and more practical than ideal. *No one gets exactly what they want.* That's how it has always been and how it will always be.

Throughout my year of study, I saw deal making up close and personal. Even the newest politicians seemed to understand the virtual demand that they "trade" their votes (and relax certain convictions) in order to get things done. I saw that compromise wasn't a virtue as much as it was a necessity.

Perhaps these observations shouldn't have been such a shocker to me at age thirty-three, but they were, and finding a conviction and voice about politics was much easier after that.

Within a few years I gravitated toward my own version of Oxford-style debates by following the debates of learned men like David Brooks and E. J. Dionne, who occupy opposing political philosophies. I found their discussions with each other to be an example of how a person could sustain convictions while finding compromise.

I also learned to *turn off* those pundits who carried the verbal and intellectual equivalent of dynamite and fire accelerant in their words.

Of course, I learned other things about politics, but accepting that policies and laws will always fall short of ideals helped me sort through the chaos of it all.

I found that politics wasn't too much different from marriage: To get through it, it's necessary to lower voices, carefully pick your battles, avoid insults and declarations of absolutes, voice *soft* lies, and *compromise, compromise, compromise.*

"Divorce," perpetual fighting, and paralysis are the unacceptable alternatives for a diverse population that wants solutions.

* * *

In March 2005, word was passed along the grapevine that then-Lieutenant General Petraeus was on the hunt for an army major working on the joint staff. The Iraqi government had selected their senior military officer (a.k.a. their chief of defense). His name was General Babakir Zibari, and Petraeus wanted to provide a US military assistant to help in the transition.

The idea of not volunteering for such an assignment may seem like an option, but no one I knew in the army saw it that way. Our personnel and performance files were sent to Petraeus's headquarters in Iraq, and then we waited. About a month later, my boss called me into his office to show me an e-mail he had received from Petraeus:

. . . [Mark] will have a tremendous vantage point, a very nonstandard mission with lots of ambiguities and drama, and an incredible opportunity to contribute. Please tell him to check in with me upon arrival.

As exciting as this was, I was more focused on the details that would affect my family. When was I leaving? What would I be doing? Where would I be working?

It took another week before I was officially notified, and even then there were few details.

When I finally met Petraeus in Iraq, I realized his earlier note about "ambiguities and drama" was an understatement. In less than five minutes, he acknowledged he wasn't quite sure how my assignment would work. He knew what he wanted, but it hadn't really been done before. He gave me some very basic guidance but told me he was leaving it to me to build a personal relationship with

Babakir.

My job was to provide Babakir with perspective on how the US Pentagon's Joint Staff was organized and run, provide 24/7 liaison to the Coalition Forces (and Petraeus), help coordinate travel (since most of it was provided by the coalition), and serve as an aide de camp (personal assistant).

As part of the coalition, it seemed odd to me that Babakir would require such hands-on assistance, but I quickly learned he had great difficulty traveling in and out of coalition checkpoints, landing zones, and airstrips. A big part of my job was to serve as the "grease" that got things done.

My duties meant I would spend 90 percent of everyday living and working where he and his staff lived and worked. I would see and hear everything they did.

The explanation and the looming unknowns had me excited but also anxious. There were infinite chances to fail, and little or no control over the things that could prevent failures. No shared culture. No shared organization values. No common language. Few shared life experiences. No shared training practices. Little agreement on how the world turns. And not a single US soldier to my left or right when I performed my work.

Nothing I had ever done in the army had prepared me for such an experience—not even my deployment to Saudi Arabia. The only way to gain the necessary skills was by doing the job and adapting as I went. The best thing I had going for me was my deep knowledge of civil and military world history—and my curiosity.

The close quarters I kept with my Iraqi partners built a level of trust that soon began to cut both ways. Sometimes my attempts to improve my US peers' understanding about coalition operations would produce heckles: "Don't go native, man. Don't let them get inside your head." I was expected to help the Iraqis understand the *coalition's* methods and plans—not the other way around.

Iraqis were equally frustrated. "Can't you make the coalition understand why we can't do it that way?"

And when it came to addressing the inevitable failings and fatalities that come with combat, Iraqi partners would frequently take out their frustrations on the closest American they could find—*an advisor* whose job included listening.

Not surprisingly, the most meaningful things I saw and heard came from Babakir himself. Whether meeting with US congressmen or chiefs of defense from dozens of other countries, visiting his family or fellow leaders around the world, discussing topics like Baghdad security-planning or his many thoughts on the US effort in Iraq, or just watching *Oprah* in his living room while drinking tea and discussing life, there seemed to be no exceptions to our interaction with each other.

In that one year, I saw more of the world and learned more about human dynamics than at any other time in my life. The experience could just as accurately be described as "my adventures with Babakir" as "my combat tour to Iraq."

Some of my experiences were better rendered at the time in journal entries and letters than they can be rendered now. In my journal, I wrote about the day I met the general:

> *I sat down with Babakir today in his ministry of defense office for our introductions. Babakir is a small man in stature. He is a Kurdish Sunni, which is the same as saying he is just a Kurd, as most Kurds seem to place ethnicity over religion. Like many Iraqis, Babakir uses his first name with his title, so he goes by "General Babakir."*
>
> *We sat on couches, and the setting was casual, but the conversation was awkward—my first with a translator. Plus, Babakir's son Arjeng (twenty years old) sat directly across from me in an office chair and stared at me like I was a rare zoo animal. I didn't mind. I figured I might be staring at him and his father the same way.*

I felt a lot of pressure to present a good first impression as we fumbled through polite small talk like we were on a forced blind date. Groping for things to talk about, Babakir's chief of staff, Jamal, brought up my experience working for our own chief of defense (General Myers) in the Pentagon. That felt even more awkward, as well as overstated. I asked if we could switch to a subject that we both knew a lot about—family.

"I am the father of three boys, which includes a set of twins," I said as I pulled pictures of Kristin and the boys from my wallet. Then I added, "I am also a twin." I could tell that really impressed him. "God smiles upon you," he said.

He told me he had nine children and explained that Kurds liked having large families. I excitedly replied that my mom was from a family of fifteen children, which seemed to impress him even more.

I noted that Babakir was a thin man and offered that my grandpa had a theory about why fathers of so many children could remain so fit. "Tell me," Babakir said as he nodded. "Well, have you ever seen a fat rooster?" I asked. He paused for a moment then laughed. Mating chickens, not work, seemed to have helped us break the ice and bridge the cultural divide.

Babakir explained that he heard many good things about me and that he was very eager to have my help. My predecessor had been gone for more than a month, and Babakir was already feeling the pain.

Sensing an appropriate close to the conversation, I asked to return to work. "No," he said, "join me for lunch." I politely declined, but he insisted, and he immediately called for his driver.

En route to Babakir's house, the realization set in that we had no translator. In our very first day together, I felt like trading in my 9mm pistol and a couple months' pay for language training. Arjeng was a reluctant English speaker, but once I convinced him that he spoke very well (and he did), he was like a godsend.

   *Babakir and I spoke about our backgrounds in the army. He
liked that I had been a soldier before becoming an officer, then
offered that it was important to personally visit soldiers, talk to
them where they worked, or to shake their hands or to kiss them.
The kissing part threw me, but I later learned its importance.
Kissing on the cheek is a sign of friendship and family in the
Middle East (and other parts of the world).*

   *At Babakir's house, he insisted I keep my boots on, but I
took them off like everyone else. (Just like at our house.) Babakir
left the room and returned a few minutes later dressed in his
traditional Kurdish Peshmerga uniform, which looked like
formal pajamas.*

   *When lunch was served, Babakir ate fast, leaving a spotless
plate in front of him long before I was done. "You eat slow," he
said. "My grandpa, the one with fifteen kids, says I eat like a
bird," I replied. And that gave him another good laugh.*

One of the first things I reviewed was Babakir's personal security detail, which consisted of seventy soldiers. That's when I met
Ali Yousef, the chief of Babakir's personal security. Ali had a larger-
than-life personality. His movie collection consisted almost entirely
of James Bond films, which appeared to serve as his only training.

Ali was loud, big hearted, and looked like the miniature
version of the Buddha, which accounts for the first Kurdish words I
learned in Iraq—*"Az berseema"* ("I am hungry"). The only English
he could speak was "not a problem," words I would gain enough
confidence to make fun of occasionally by replying, "No, Ali. *Big
fucking problem.*"

As funny as this was to me at the time, I realized that "not a
problem" and "I am hungry" would not suffice in a security crisis.
We needed to be able to communicate with more than smiles
and grunts.

Within the first week of meeting Babakir, I decided I needed to learn Kurdish. Arabic was an option, but Kurdish was Babakir's native tongue, and I was always surrounded by family and friends ready to teach me.

Within three months, they said I could carry on a conversation with relative competence, but I always felt just as apprehensive as Arjeng during our first week together.

About three months into my assignment with Babakir, I sent an e-mail home that showed a growing sense of comfort with my discomfort.

Kristin—

Well, considering my dilemma with the "runs" this week, one would think the flu was in season. But it must be the Iraqi food. In any case, my digestive system is in chaos.

Babakir and the gang heard about it and had a grand time busting my chops and laughing at my expense. (I laughed right along with them.) Intestinal problems are a pretty common thing among the Iraqis. And since they don't use toilet paper, I've learned to carry it the same way I carry my weapon and ammo.

Speaking of food, we had lunch the other day with the soldiers of the Iraqi 6th Division. When we arrived, the tables were already filled with huge beds of rice, sprinkled with almonds, chick peas, and what looked like raisins. Huge chunks of lamb (still on the bone) were buried in the rice. Suddenly I was aware that the raisins were not raisins. They were dead flies that had apparently been "captured" during preparation.

Aside from the flies, the food actually looked and smelled pretty darn good. Too bad my face didn't communicate that message. The Iraqi sitting next to me said, "What the matter my friend, why you are not eating."

"There aren't enough flies on this food."

"The flies, they make you strong . . . from the inside," he

replied.

"You mean from getting sick so often that your immune system gets stronger?" I said with a smile.

"Yes, yes. Come on now, eat," he said without even looking up from his plate. "Just pick them out." He spoke about it like we were talking about picking out mushrooms.

Still, as disgusting as it was to me, this was their life, and they weren't exactly asking me to eat poison. I grabbed a spoon and dug right in (minding the flies). Wasn't too bad, and the meat was actually delicious. Still, the flies.

Afterward we enjoyed some mouthwatering baklava and a nice warm Pepsi to wash it all down. Mmm. Ain't nothin' like a warm refreshing Pepsi in 120-degree heat.

Speaking of the heat. You know it's bad when you start wishing for a return to the low 100s. The temp is sure to climb to above 120 degrees this summer. This stuff just takes your breath away. Every time I breathe it in I think back to our days in Minnesota and recall the days when it was so cold you could feel your lungs freeze as you breathed in the air—but at least you could breathe it. The heat here is suffocating. May sound stupid, but now I know how SpongeBob and Patrick feel in that movie (the one the boys watch all the time) when they're being dried out under that sun lamp.

Love,

Me

And it wasn't just the physical discomfort I was getting used to. It was moral discomfort, too, as I told Kristin in another letter.

Just like my deployment to Saudi Arabia, it is hard—really hard—to manage the personal biases I have as an American. You know how much I read and how much I try to stay plugged in, and yet I realize I don't have a clue. I can't help but imagine what it might be like among soldiers who don't make any effort to understand these surroundings.

Every day I am subjected to the blunt distinction of these two worlds in a dozen little ways:

In the morning, I make my way through the embassy to a breakfast that reminds me of royal dining halls. Of course, this has much more to do with the fact that the army contracts out its food service, which requires strict cleanliness and preparation standards. But still. It's a sight. The amount of food that is thrown away every day is grotesque when I think about the starvation occurring in some of the surrounding neighborhoods.

That starvation is NOT our problem, but it still bothers me.

Then I make my way out to the parking lot, which is full of brand-new Ford Explorers and dozens of armored Ford Expeditions and Chevy Suburbans armed to the teeth.

On my way, I pass the PX food court where, if you've not managed to stuff your face enough with the free food, you can willy-nilly spend your bucks and gorge on Burger King or the Pizza Inn. I usually pick up a copy of the Stars and Stripes newspaper, and my "favorite" days are when there's a story about Michael Jackson on the cover. (Not.)

Within minutes I am transported to what I like to call "the Wild" and things change dramatically. These guys [Iraqis] drink out of the same cups, drink water from the tap (which is not safe), take shits without toilet paper, drive old vehicles that barely run, leave the safety of the Green Zone every afternoon, and then brave what's called the "Assassins' Gate" every morning on their way into work.

Iraqis accept this dichotomy without much complaint—until they taste what we have. Let me tell you, they don't need to be convinced that one is better than the other. Forget sports, entertainment, business, modern medicines, or material goods. *They just want the basics. How basic? I'll just give you one example that shook my senses:*

Colonel Jamal, one of the Iraqi officers, told me last week that he needed some time off. He wanted two weeks, which was too long by any standard, especially for the position he held with Babakir. Plus, he always seemed distracted and a little scatterbrained. I thought it was laziness. I'm used to hearing lame excuses, so I was ready for a whopper when I finally asked, "Why do you need to go?" He said that he needed to go to Syria to get his family and bring them back to Baghdad now that he had secured a home in the Green Zone for them.

I didn't need to hear any more, but he continued the story and I listened.

He had been in the Iraqi Army all of his life, but never in positions of great responsibility or command. He married and had three children, all of whom are still under the age of fourteen. He learned English by watching American movies, and speaks it well. When US forces crossed into Iraq in March 2003, he was serving in Baghdad and clearly remembers when the bombs started falling. When the war ended and the army ceased to exist, he melted into the population like everyone else. Then he received word that the coalition was looking for a "few good men." His low rank, modest background, and English-speaking skills made him an easy pick.

He and his family began receiving death threats immediately—two or three of them over several months. He ignored them. Then his neighbor and their entire family were killed. Jamal panicked. He immediately packed up his family and left Baghdad without telling anyone.

Shortly after his arrival to the northern Iraqi city of Mosul, an insurgent "checkpoint" stopped a group of a dozen or so vehicles. Everyone was brought to a small clearing and interrogated to see who worked for the coalition. One poor

*bastard had some sort of coalition identification on him. (Jamal
said that thankfully he did not.) The insurgents forced everyone
to look at the young man, announced that what was about to
happen would happen to them as well if they worked for the
coalition, and then he proceeded to cut the guy's head off.*

*Jamal explained, with a disturbing calm, that the man " . . .
shook like a chicken. And the blood, it shoot everywhere. Right in
front of my kids, man," he said with misty eyes.*

*He immediately went home, packed up all his belongings, and
moved his family to Syria, where they've been ever since. "I have no
other family; I have no other reason to live. No mother, no father,
no brothers or sisters, no aunts or uncles . . . my wife and kids, they
are all I have, you know?" God, I can only imagine.*

*In sharing this daily perspective about my observations of two
different worlds, I want to be clear. This is not a "bash America
and its ways" fest, or "this is why we need to be out of Iraq."
I'm merely pointing out a personal struggle with perspective
as I live in two very different places each day. Our sports and
entertainment, as well as our business sense and preoccupation
with material goods, are just so out-of-this-world different from
this place. It's hard to balance.*

And then there were other moments when the worlds seemed
to come together as one. From my journal:

*Today is Saturday in the States, but "Sunday" in Iraq. In Islam,
Friday is the holy day of the week and the first day of their
weekend; thus Saturday is their Sunday.*

*I arranged a dinner last night at Babakir's house between
Babakir and Brigadier General Cris Anstey, a new Aussie general
assigned to MNSTC-I. It was quite entertaining. As usual,
Babakir had me sit next to him at the table. (I have dinner or
a late lunch at his home about three or four times per week, but*

usually with his staff in the kitchen. I prefer sitting with them and learning about how things work behind the scenes.)

They brought the food to the table, and we all dug right in. This was Anstey's first week in the country and his first informal meeting with Babakir. Anstey looked across the table and commented in his thick Aussie accent, "Ahh, couscous! I love couscous." [Pronounced "coos coos."] The table erupted in laughter. Couscous is apparently a mixture of barley and meat—in Australia. Arabs and Kurds eat the same thing, but they don't call it couscous, and for good reason. Apparently a word pronounced "coos coos" means "pussy" in Arabic (or Kurdish), and I'm not referring to the cat.

The subject really broke the ice at the table and unavoidably started a discussion about women. Babakir commented about how things in the Middle East were not much different than anywhere else when it came to humor about some women. Then he told a joke:

There once was an Arab man who kept a picture of his mother-in-law on an end table at his home in Germany. A visiting stranger commented that the Arab must really love his mother-in-law to have her picture on such a prominent place in his home. The Arab replied that his mother-in-law was actually back in his home country, but that he didn't miss her at all because he really didn't like her. The visitor was stunned and asked about the obvious contradiction. The Arab replied that what he really loved and missed was his home country, but he kept that picture visible so he would be reminded of what came with the deal.

After dinner, we sat in the living room and had tea while Babakir scrolled through the TV channels. He stopped at Oprah and set the remote down. The show was in English, but had Arabic script running across the bottom of the screen. I wanted to pinch myself.

Oprah's guest was Shania Twain, and Twain had just

finished talking about her childhood, how poor she was growing up, and how badly she wished she could share her present-day experiences with her deceased mother. She cried as she told the story, and Babakir was clearly moved by it all.

I later learned that Oprah was a bit of a favorite in Babakir's home, and once again I was humbled by the strange way the world seemed to turn. Oprah in Iraq? Why not?

By the time I took my second trip to the Kurdish region of Iraq with Babakir, it became clear to me that he (and his family) considered me to be much more than just an American army officer. They bragged to everyone they knew that I was a Kurdish-American. Babakir's family prepared a feast that took several women three days to prepare.

All the men sat in a circle at the Kurdish kitchen table (the floor). When we sat, Babakir tapped the floor next to him and nodded for me to sit next to him. He treated me like one of his children, and I truly felt like one of them.

That evening, Babakir received a dozen guests into his living room, and I was invited to join them. I wore the traditional Kurdish dress of the Peshmerga soldier (the formal-looking pajamas I'd seen on Babakir six months prior), a gift that Babakir's cousin, Otto, had made for me. The sight drew excitement and surprise from the men, all of whom were dressed the same way, and giggles from the women, who sat separate from the men.

I took up a spot on the couch, and conversations sprung up all around. I felt very uncomfortable wearing their Peshmerga uniform. I hadn't earned it. I suggested that perhaps I should change, and I was unanimously yelled at to sit down. They would not have it. I was Kurdish, as far as they were concerned.

Babakir suddenly announced to the people in the room in Kurdish, "This man, he's like a son to me." He smiled longingly at me and then told the group some quick stories about our adventures in Baghdad and in Germany. I replied I was nothing more than a good-natured mule—and not always good natured, which really was the truth. Babakir clicked his tongue and scolded me. "You are not mule," he said in clear English. "And you are good man."

More small talk broke out, but much of it focused on me, "the blue-eyed, blond-haired Kurdish Peshmerga," many of them said as they laughed with pride. The women echoed the comment, saying I looked very handsome. I broke into conversation using my Kurdish, and the room just lit up.

Under Saddam Hussein, speaking Kurdish was against the law, which effectively made it a dying language—like a dialect of Native American Cherokee, it didn't have much use outside the tribe. By speaking it, it seemed I was touching the very soul of every man and woman in the room, and they weren't shy telling me how much it meant to them.

Babakir again interrupted the group of men and asked me what color headdress I would decide to wear: red or black. I asked him what the difference was, and he told me red represented the tribes of the Barzani family, while black represented the tribes of his own Zibari family.

Babakir had taught me long before that the Barzani tribe initiated the insurrection against the Ottoman Empire in the early 1900s. And for more than thirty years, Mustafa Barzani was the political and military leader of the Kurdish revolution against successive Iraqi regimes in Baghdad. Although the Kurds were never able to establish a nation for themselves, Mustafa is widely considered the George Washington of the Kurdish people. In short, custom demanded deference to the Barzani family.

I had an idea, then, that the gathered men expected to hear me say Barzani, particularly if Babakir had presumably taught me properly. But instead I answered with what I firmly believed, "I would wear the black, of course." The men politely chuckled and whispered to one another. Babakir clicked his tongue and in a hushed voice said in clear English, "Nooo, Mark, nooo. Barzani is better." He said it as if I had just ignorantly insulted him and everyone in the room.

The man sitting next to me asked in Kurdish with a smile, "*Zibari, Boo?*" ("Why Zibari?") I answered, "*Barzani? Ava Boscha.*" (The word *boscha* means many things depending on the tone and context; in this case, it meant "better.")

Every man in the room sighed with relief and tilted his head back, "*Ahh, boscha, boscha,*" they mumbled. Even Babakir smiled approvingly.

That's when I set the hook and yelled loudly with a big smile on my face, "*But Zibari, zur Boscha!*" ("Zibari is much better!") And I quickly explained, "*Babakir Zibari, Bobymin. Boo ch'nia Zibari?*" ("Babakir Zibari is my father. Why wouldn't I pick Zibari?")

The room erupted in laughter and slaps on the knee.

My reply was spontaneous, and it was somewhat taboo for a foreigner to say, but it just naturally occurred to me after being with Babakir for so long, if I were a Kurd at all, I was a *Zibari* Kurd.

Numerous Zibari family members later told me they thought it one of the most clever things someone could say in such a situation. What I had failed to do by custom, I more than made up for in principle and character, and everyone seemed to respect that as much or more than tradition.

I heard Babakir tell that story a dozen times in the months that followed, and each time he told it he laughed, and his guests laughed with him. As casual as I thought that exchange had been, I think it defined our relationship.

Not long after, Babakir declared he was going to start calling me by a Kurdish name he had come up with for me: Sherzod Zibari, which he said meant "son of lion," his American-born son.

(My Aussie friends wasted no time in clarifying to our coalition comrades that Sherzod really meant "nutsack.")

★ ★ ★

When the time came for me to leave Iraq after twelve months, Babakir asked then-Lieutenant General Martin Dempsey if I could stay. Dempsey and I spoke, and I took a passive approach.

I didn't think I was irreplaceable, but I did recognize the importance and practicality of staying. After all, General Casey's aide had been with him for more than two years. The reason for that long relationship was obvious; they had a connection that was personal and preferred in the relative chaos of Iraq.

Babakir and I shared the same relationship, and he naturally wanted to keep that. I respected that desire and said I would stay, but I wasn't going to ask for it—not with a wife and you boys waiting for me at home.

Babakir wrote a letter explaining why he wanted to keep me:

He is aggressive in his work and he tells me hard truths, but he is also humble, his advice is diplomatic, and he is sensitive to culture. Mark has been like a son to me, and he is the first American officer that I know who has learned the Kurdish language . . . All of these reasons make him very, very effective, and these are the reasons why I do not want to lose him.

When the decision was made to send me home, Babakir accepted it with grace and wrote an embarrassingly flattering letter recommending promotion, recognition, and the best evaluation Dempsey could write. Babakir wrote, in part, "There were so many officers who served with me who had higher ranks than Mark by many years, but . . . he was the best one among them."

Babakir's personal letters about my work with him are still more valuable to me than any military recognition I received from my year in Iraq.

He threw me a farewell feast fit for a king. Generals Dempsey and Chiarelli joined us for dinner, but even more impressive was the attendance of the Iraqi senior military command. They were all there: the chief of the Iraqi Army, General Abdul Qadir Obeidi; the chief of the Iraqi Air Force, General Kemal Barzanji; and Iraq's deputy chief of defense, General Nasier Abadi.

We had lived together, eaten together, mourned together, and traveled together. I knew them, and I felt they knew me as much as any American soldiers I had ever met.

* * *

Meekness is another word for *humility*. But in MacArthur's context it means "gentleness" of true strength, and he clarifies it elsewhere when he says, "to learn to stand up in the storm, but to have compassion on those who fall."

When my cancer battle started in 2010, I assumed everyone I knew would be willing and able to mirror my strength and attitude back to me. I thought they would appreciate and—from the way I received the news of the diagnosis—understand my decision to return to work despite the cancer still growing inside me and support my plan to manage my pain without medication.

Nearly everyone said they admired it, but few said they could comprehend how it was possible, let alone advisable.

The medical professionals questioned me often on my ability to tackle such a crushing change to my life and routine, which was pronounced in light of my profession as a soldier. Doctors and nurses repeatedly reassured me there was no shame in taking antidepressants, as if I might be holding back a bit about how I was *really* doing.

"What you've experienced is really as serious and as nasty as it gets," my surgeon told me. He didn't know many people who could take it the way I seemed to be taking it.

Far from being flattered, I was frustrated. I didn't like being singled out, and it still bugs me when I am, because the implication is that I'm not normal—a message that, if delivered often enough, makes me feel isolated, not exceptional.

Examples of my "abnormality"? I packed my own wounds. I insisted on giving my fevers time to indicate their course before running to the ER or asking for antibiotics. And when pain or fear or sadness struck, I sought out not drugs but *perspective* to help me laugh or find the blessings around me to help balance the scales. I nicknamed my two interventional radiologists Oscar and Felix (from the TV show *The Odd Couple*) and joked with them or offered advice—under sedation—during my procedures. I reflected on the fact that twelve years ago there was no treatment at all for what I had and I could be dead already. And I often refused pain medication in favor of a clear head.

Of course, being so involved and self-reliant was sometimes hard work, and it didn't always give me hope about improved health. But I didn't think it was all *that* difficult when I considered the fact that every bad thing I was experiencing was going to happen whether I was involved or not.

Being involved made me feel more in control.

In time, I came to realize I needed to be gentler and more compassionate about how I addressed people who said they were inspired by or in disbelief about my choices.

One way I tried to turn my frustration into encouragement was to help others absorb what I considered to be a truth about hardship: "*Someone always has it worse than you do.*"

I explained to family and friends how an eleven-year-old-girl up the street from us burned herself with a curling iron and contracted strep A. She was dead in a week. That same week—Thanksgiving week—a man was driving up a county road just a few miles from our house when a deer stepped out in front of his car, went through the windshield, and killed him instantly. No goodbyes. No reflections. Gone.

These two stories were from just one day in time and within a half mile from where I lived. And there were just as many examples of people who didn't die, but lived in a pain and misery that seemed much worse than mine.

You don't have to speak in the abstract about the blessings of life when we're surrounded by such examples. When you remember how many others have it worse—or who suffer the same pain you do—you just can't help but feel blessed or encouraged as you contend with the Bufords in your own life.

✷ ✷ ✷

Few subjects tickle your soul and your sense of humility like faith, religion, the meaning of life, and the *thought* of what will come when we die. In August 2010, while I was lying in my hospital bed like a cut-open deer carcass, comments and questions about these subjects came more frequently than they had in all my life, and they haven't slowed up since.

The vast majority of people were social, as in, "I'll pray for your family" or "God be with you and your family."

But a good number of well-wishers sought to provide something more than social. No matter which religion these people practiced, the theme of the sentiment, both explicit and implied, was, "I want to make sure you get into heaven."

I'm certain love and good intentions fueled their efforts, but there was nothing humble, open-minded, or meek about it. There was a specific prescription, and I needed to recite the magic words, or I was "not going to be saved."

Even in combat, most of my adult experiences with afterlife discussions were little more than coded talk about who might go to hell and who might get to heaven. Now there was nothing coded about it. Fear, *not hope*, led these discussions.

Noah once overheard me patiently responding to a persistent stranger on the topic and asked, "Why didn't you just hang up, Dad?" That's a tough question to answer in one sentence, but I answered honestly, "Because I learn a little about myself when I have such conversations."

And that's what I find myself reflecting upon here as I read MacArthur's words: To focus less on how, why, and what *others* might say or do and focus more on how, why, and what *you* will say or do.

✷ ✷ ✷

It's tempting to read MacArthur's words and see three separate proposals: To seek humility, find true wisdom with an open mind, and to discover the meekness of true strength. But he is only making one proposal—that you should be humble and recognize what you don't know or understand. In that context, you'll find and appreciate the other two.

When MacArthur spoke to that room of cadets in 1962, he warned there was no way he could communicate all that his words fully meant. In my view, there is no other subject where that idea is truer than with religion. It is in that spirit that I propose to be a bit more direct in passing along what my experiences have taught me.

First, the only thing I am 100 percent certain about with faith, the meaning of life, and the concept of the afterlife is that sooner or later, they are subjects you will face. Please trust me when I tell you it is best to consider your spirituality throughout your life—that's what it's for, after all—rather than late in life or under duress.

Second, try to imagine faith as a dog with religion as its tail. Religion is what you use to practice your faith, not the other way around. At least consider that we're all praying to and finding inspiration from the same creator, regardless of our chosen prophet or practice. I think this thinking takes as much or more faith than does grimly holding onto the notion that only one can be correct.

Above all, discussion of religion should never involve criticizing others about theirs; rather, it should be about reflecting on your own religion and being humble with how you treat yourself and others.

You know my religion, and religion is vitally *important, but I want to leave you with an explicit example I hope will reward you the way it has me—not only with knowledge and wisdom, but with a love and understanding that has truly made life worth living.*[10]

One day with Babakir in Iraq, I was expressing frustration over something someone did during a recent trip and I made a familiar exclamation, "My God, you've got to be kidding me."

Babakir stopped what he was doing, grabbed my arm, looked me square in the eyes, and said, "Mark, why you always say 'my God'? Not your God. Our God."

---

10. I encourage you to read *Speaking Christian* by Marcus Borg, which offers a more humble approach to how Christians should consider speaking. Also, Rob Bell's *Love Wins*, another fairly humble and incredibly thought-provoking work that asks questions and poses issues that may seem new, but are as old as Christianity itself. And since Bell is praised as well as criticized for his observations, consider reading *God Wins* by Mark Galli, which offers a fairly even-handed response to Bell's book. Finally, consider reading *The Evolution of God* from nontheologian Robert Wright, who underscores the importance of faith over practice of faith.

CHAPTER SEVEN

. . . To be serious, yet never to take yourself too seriously; to cry, but also to laugh.

January 2012

Buford's abscess continued to persist as it had the previous four months, and I spent Christmas Eve in the hospital following the failure of a fourth experiment in as many months. What was once only a bile leak now involved mashed food escaping from my intestine. The hole was getting bigger.

The excruciating pain was bad enough, but what I found far worse was the necessary routine involved in each hospital visit with doctors and nurses. It didn't matter how well I knew my own case; they were often obliged to follow their protocols. And I *rejected* protocols for their own sake:

What's that shot? Heprin? No, thank you. I stay active, so blood clotting is not an issue.

What's with the Protonix? I take Aciphex, and I brought it with me. What do you mean I can't take it because it wasn't prescribed here?

Why are you taking blood again? Routine? Unless you're checking something specific, no.

Why are we doing a CT scan? If my treatment will remain unchanged [and it usually did], *no, we're not doing a CT scan.*

If a test or procedure didn't make sense or couldn't be explained as being applicable to any symptom or condition I was experiencing, I refused it.

The second day in the hospital, my surgeon instructed my nurses to take me off my chemo. My weight was down to 137 pounds, I was on my second day without food, and they already had me on a bowel cleanse for a fifth experiment they wanted to perform.

What does it hurt for me to continue taking the medication that's keeping the cancer asleep?

In short, their answer was nothing more than "protocol."

"You know, a few days off the chemo probably won't matter, anyway."

Probably won't matter? Really?! Well, shit, if you're that certain, then how can a dumbass like me possibly argue with that logic?

I lost it.

When the nurse retreated from the room and I was alone with my thoughts, I felt a wave of emotion sweep over me, as if months of pain, misery, and helplessness came pouring into my mind all at once—*great* anger, and then an uncertainty and fear that seized my throat in a vice. I felt as if I were being treated like a five-year-old, and I suddenly felt like one. I burst into tears and punched the bed with both fists. Rather than argue with the tears, I let the emotion flow.

After taking an emotional knee for a few minutes, it seemed easier to turn my focus back to what needed to be done. I was polite, but I peppered my feedback to the medical team with "effen-heimers" to impress upon them that I was and would continue to be a part of the team. I understood if other people didn't make a fuss, but *I* was not them. (I had Kristin bring my chemo from home, and I took it without their permission.)

They sent me home a few days later with my latest Buford appliance—a drainage tube with a small balloon that was inflated inside the intestine. The intent was to stop up the hole, which I now affectionately referred to as the "bullet hole."

Less than a week later, I flew to St. Louis to deliver a motivational speech to about thirty veterans of the armed forces as they began their fellowships with The Mission Continues, a nonprofit organization established by former Navy Seal Eric Greitens. (The idea: Challenge post-9/11 veterans to serve and inspire others in communities across America and help them find the same sense of purpose they had when they were in uniform.)

The night before the speech, the laws of physics somehow forced that balloon to tear through the intestine and lodge itself in my abdominal muscle.

I gritted my teeth the next morning, delivered my remarks, and then flew home and checked myself into the hospital, which turned into a weeklong stay.

When doctors told me a feeding tube was now unavoidable, I again waited until I was left with my own thoughts, took a knee, and just let the tears flow. The idea of not being able to eat food— to be denied something so fundamentally joyful and social and *normal*—was overwhelming.

Since I was a little boy, I couldn't remember crying as often as I had in that past year. As a young man, maybe I'd cried a dozen times in fifteen years, with great sorrow at the funerals of my grandparents and with joy at my wedding and the births of you boys.

Now I saw profound sadness and joy in everything. As a friend of mine jokes, I cried at card tricks and supermarket openings.

I also laughed as much as I ever did before—and I've always laughed a lot.

Laughter has come naturally to me during hardships and crisis, but I think it would be misleading to say that's just who I am. Humor is a coping mechanism of choice, and it had always seemed to reward me, so I chose it a lot.

All my life, I've sought out perspectives that could wring laughter from pain, and I got an early start with an alcoholic family and a shower-room bully. Finding and sharing humor with dignity, grace, and even respect for those who see no humor in a crappy situation takes work so it doesn't come off as being crude. (We've all seen the devastating result of a poorly timed or poorly handled joke.)

Over time, I've learned to console myself and others in the proportional relationship: the shittier the situation, the funnier the story.

✷ ✷ ✷

Oftentimes, finding humor not only produces a good feeling, it helps me communicate—*particularly with three young boys*. Humor has helped us get into topics we might otherwise have just drifted past.

Within weeks of arriving home from the hospital after the big surgery, I commented to you all that I was about as useful as the family cat, Abby. All I did was eat, sleep, and defecate. At least the cat had a litter box and didn't really smell as she strolled around the house. Even if I didn't find the comparison funny, you boys did, and it helped us talk about all sorts of related topics.

Two years after the surgery, my digestive system and liver have been permanently damaged, and the smell that still comes out of me can only be described as unholy. Anyone who has been on a hunting or camping trip and experienced the effects of a changed diet might begin to relate.

In addition to the foul-smelling gas, my drainage bags are portable sacks of shit-smelling juice. They accompany me everywhere and produce an odor as permanent as cat urine or skunk spray.

Sometimes Kristin follows me around the house, making sure the gas hasn't turned into a liquid. Nothing contains the smell (we've tried).

The cat doesn't disagree with the comparison. Prior to the surgery, Abby always wanted to sit on my lap; I always pushed her off and said I thought her butt stunk. Now she doesn't come anywhere near me. She usually walks by, pauses, looks up at me, then continues on her way. I can't help but hear what she's thinking during that pause, "You know what? The stink ain't worth it. Fuck the scratch and your warm lap. I'll go rub my neck on the cement stairs and lie in the sunlight."

For Kristin and all of you, I've concluded that all I can do is apologize and laughingly accept Kristin's declaration that we're going to light the furniture ablaze someday in a spectacular back-yard bonfire. Kristin and I still chuckle about the time she lovingly told me I was on my own with administering a home enema kit.

The addition of a feeding tube a year later only furthered the cat analogy when, like Abby, I was not allowed to eat table food. In fact, when it came to food, I was more like those finicky cats who prance in TV commercials.

Food from a bag? Pshaw. My food can only come from a can.

★ ★ ★

Sometimes it helps to give yourself something else to cry about.

When I was about fourteen years old, I stubbed my toe so badly that it bled. Somehow my dad and I crossed paths in my crying stupor. He expressed his concern, rubbed my back, and told me it would be okay, and then he suddenly punched me in the leg.

"How does your toe feel now?" he said with a laugh.

His technique may sound sadistic, and it wasn't the first time I'd experienced it, but it worked. He had literally given me something else to cry (or at least think) about.

When you think your life is bad or unfair, take a trip to the children's hospital or the VA hospital or a local mental ward to give yourself a proverbial punch in the leg. It won't change *anything* about your circumstances, but it will damn sure have you looking at your own hardships differently.

A buddy of mine, John Kriesel, lost both of his legs in Iraq and spent more than a year in the hospital and rehab. He commented to me, "Thank God I don't have what you have."

You will always find someone who has it worse than you do.

✯ ✯ ✯

The one thing you have to know about cancer is that it's shitty—*literally*. From surgeries and chemo comes everything from constipation to diarrhea, and from smelly to outright disaster, both in public and at home. Personal dignity is what's at stake, and if you can't find *just a little* humor in the unavoidable existence of it all, dignity is what I think gets lost quickly.

As often happens in life, the most miserable, humiliating, indescribable moment turned out to be the funniest of all.

Just a few weeks into my home recovery, I was still on a high dose of Dilaudid (morphine times ten), which put my digestive tract to sleep along with my pain. Hours of immense pain in my upper abdomen turned into a fever and chills, so we went to the ER.

The doc ordered a CT scan and discovered a partially obstructed bowel at the top of my intestine near the stomach. Though I'd had regular bowel movements, the ER doc said obstructions still occur.

What happened next can only be described as professional torture in the name of medicine—waterboarding, in reverse.

They rolled me down the hall and put me up on an X-ray table, which seemed more like a big countertop. The thought of getting my first enema while I was in so much pain and whacked out on drugs caused enough anxiety by itself; it only got worse after I realized it was my lab technician's first day on the job.

I stared in disbelief when she rolled in the IV pole with the gallon-size bag of fluid that would be pumped up my rear end. Their emphasis on how warm the fluid was did *not* brighten my spirits.

After the prep, which included inflating a balloon inside my rectum to keep the fluid from coming out, the doctor entered the room. I bit my lip to keep from bursting into laughter and considered the possibility I was hallucinating.

The small Asian man was dressed in a black, plastic-looking gown tied so tightly around his body, it looked as if he wrapped himself in it.

The only light in the room came from the monitor in front of him, which made his gown sparkle; his teeth shine bright white; and his small, round-rimmed glasses look like sunglasses. A dark hat tied around his forehead completed the dress. He looked like a mad scientist version of *The Karate Kid*'s Mr. Miyagi.

He was friendly but very direct, which told me he probably had a lot of experience with patients who did not relish the idea of having a gallon of fluid pumped up their exit ramp. He studied the CT images with furl-browed intensity. "Oh, you got lotta poo up dare."

I told him I had had regular bowel movements, but I may as well have been talking to the wall. "Yep, lotta poo dare . . . not nowmal dare."

Mr. Miyagi ordered the techs to release the fluid, and the only thing that seemed to be missing was a maniacal laugh after he said it.

The pain of that fluid was *immediately* unbearable, and the back pressure pushed yellow ooze out from Buford and onto my stomach. "Twenty-fi percen dare . . . doing good." About thirty seconds later, "Fity percent now," and right then, the entire X-ray tabletop started to move. They hadn't prepared me for this part of the freak show, and being high on drugs didn't help.

I was now inverted on the table at 45 degrees, with my feet up in the air and head close to the floor.

"Oh God, let me off this ride," I yelled, half-joking and half-serious. The pain was so intense, I couldn't help but moan pathetically.

"Seventy-fi percen dare now." The poltergeist-propelled table tipped back forward, and then back again.

"Niney-fi percen . . . all mo dare now." About thirty seconds later, he repeated, "Niney-fi percen."

"Hey!" I yelled. "You already said 95 percent!" I could hear soft chuckles in the room from the techs, but the doc didn't skip a beat, even as I howled like a 140-pound baby.

"Niney-six . . . niney seven . . . "—longer break—"niney eight . . . gotta get all way up dare . . . believe me . . . best way to clean bowel right here. You hol for fi or ten minute, and you do great."

I don't think I ever wanted to hurt a man more than I wanted to hurt that doctor right then.

Finally Miyagi finished. The tech backed out a little of the fluid and then suggested I be allowed to go to the toilet. "No," I told her. "If keeping it in for five minutes is going to help get the mud off the walls, then leave me be." And she did.

What followed then, and all the rest of that day, cannot be adequately described by words. My poor rear end. Friends asked if I felt any better. *I didn't even know what that meant.* All I knew was that when the pain was gone, I laughed until I cried each of the three times I shared that story over the next two days, and *that* felt wonderful.

☆ ☆ ☆

When you work for the most senior military officer in the armed forces, there's a vital requirement to take things seriously and a natural tendency to take yourself too seriously as well. But throughout my career, I've found there is usually a time, a place, and a way to ensure the air doesn't get too stuffy at work.

Most people working in the Pentagon put in a normal workday. But if you work on the personal staff of a senior leader, life is very different. And it doesn't get much busier than working for the chairman of the Joint Chiefs of Staff. I left the house at 4:30 a.m., and most days I didn't get home until after you boys were in bed. It was a grueling, tireless task, but I loved it.

Every day when I went into my Pentagon office, I walked past large photos of Secretary of Defense Rumsfeld, Chairman of the Joint Chiefs of Staff General Myers, and Vice Chairman of the Joint Chiefs of Staff General Pace. In a public affairs office, such pictures are like trophies, a photographic acknowledgement of these leaders' importance.

One of the photos showed General Pace addressing a town hall, with Rumsfeld standing off to the side, staring at Pace with an intense gaze. Everyone in the office got a good chuckle when I added a paper bubble above the picture of Rumsfeld's head with the words "Damn, he's good!"

The next day the photo was gone. We later found out General Pace had taken it down. Perhaps I had gone too far.

Within hours, we had the full story. Pace loved the humorous reference, and he had taken the photo to show Rumsfeld. Rumsfeld loved it, too, and immediately showed it to some visiting dignitaries. Pace brought the photo back down to his office to return it to us, but it disappeared again. Rumsfeld had sent for it, because he wanted to keep it. He even sent Pace a personal note about it and had him come to his office to pose with it.

Today, I have the photo of the two of them holding my mocked-up photo with two big smiles on their faces, as well as the "snowflake" memo Rumsfeld wrote to Pace that day.

TO: Gen Pete Pace
FROM: Donald Rumsfeld [with handwritten initials]
SUBJECT: "Damn, he's good!" Photo

I see you've made the wall in my office under Karzai and Musharaff. Good company. All source intel reports a leading member of the "Pete Pace Maximum Leader" Committee put the poster in its [current] place—sometimes you have got to take matters into your own hands, I guess.

And, yes, you are good.
DHR

Rumsfeld was referring to the fact that Pace was a contender to replace General Myers as the nation's top military officer. Shortly after this incident, General Pace *was* selected to be the new chairman, and he later sent me the Rumsfeld "snowflake" with a personal inscription handwritten in the lower margin:

Mark,

> *Never let a promising career stand in the way of a good joke!!*
> *With Respect,*

Peter Pace
General, USMC (Ret)
16th CJCS

Just like the "duck walk" so many years ago, this small gesture—in this case, a well-placed bit of humor amid the chaos of life—managed to generate more positive attention than I ever bargained for.

★ ★ ★

My time in Iraq contained as many absurd moments as Joseph Heller's book *Catch-22*.

There was the crowded flight with Babakir, in which he was randomly asked to intercede in a quarrel between a British and an Arab traveler. Or the time my Ford Explorer pickup truck (with coalition checkpoint credentials) had been stolen from a landing zone, which I feared had been turned into a car bomb. Or, against my better judgment and at Babakir's insistence, there was the time he and I drove through Baghdad in a rusted-out, late-model car with no escort, no weapons, and no protective gear.

Then there was the night in Iraq when I'd just flopped into my bed after a very long day and I heard a combination of popping corn and hail bouncing off the roof of the trailer.

My roommate turned off the TV, and I shot up from the bed. When we lived on Fort Leonard Wood, Kristin and I could hear hundreds of soldiers shooting their weapons on "range row" several miles down the road from family housing. *This* noise, however, sounded like tens of thousands of people firing weapons from every single direction, *which included the "thump, thump, thump" of heavy machine guns.*

Iraq had beaten Syria in a soccer game.

We learned the next day that the "celebration" killed forty-three Baghdad citizens.

In terms of sheer density of absurdity, however, nothing approached my adventure as an accidental "gunrunner."

During a social gathering of all the advisors to the Iraqi Ministry of Defense, I received a call on my cell phone. It was Babakir's cousin, Kurdo, and I could hear Babakir speaking in the background. He needed help. Several trucks had arrived at a coalition checkpoint loaded with weapons for the Iraqi Army, and they weren't allowed to pass.

One of the senior advisors, an Aussie general, said he didn't think I should help. "No, mate, we need to get the Iraqi J4"—logistics—"involved in this. Just stay out of it." Though I fully agreed, it was 5:30 p.m. on a Friday afternoon, and this was a personal request from the top regarding a coalition checkpoint issue.

I walked over and explained the situation to the officer who advised the Iraqi Ministry of Defense on logistics issues. Instead of helping, he vented his frustration about working with the Iraqis, then offered this useless advice: "I think this is a prime example of where we need to let . . . them . . . fail." Besides, he explained, there were no real procedures to deal with this.

"Wow, that's brilliant," I said. "So that'll teach them not to use procedures that don't exist."

I had no idea how I was going to accomplish the task, but doing nothing was not an option. Knowing Kurdo was already en route, I broke into a trot across the rooftop where we were gathered, stepped through the door, and bounded down the narrow staircase.

BAM! The sound of a bat hitting a ball.

My lower body shot forward, and I did a backflip as everything in my hands flew across the room and I landed on the cement floor below.

I had failed to clear the available headroom, and my forehead struck the landing above.

I immediately heard two officers standing just a few steps away yell out, "*Ohhholy* shit!" They rushed over to me as I tried to sit up. "You better take a moment," one of them said.

"I'm fine," I replied. "I just need a minute here—I know that must have looked bad, but my pride is hurt more than anything else." The knot on my forehead and the dripping blood didn't make me very convincing.

"You don't know that, bud. You may need to see someone for that," he replied. I sat there patiently, but my focus was still on the checkpoint. I sat a few minutes to humor my Good Samaritan friends then jumped up, thanked the officers for their assistance, and bolted out the door.

When I arrived at Checkpoint 18 on the far-west side of the Green Zone, it felt like I'd stepped into another dimension. The checkpoint was run by Russian-Georgian troops colocated with Iraqi soldiers and a hodgepodge of interpreters who could speak Russian and Arabic, but not English. Kurdo could speak English and Kurdish, but not Arabic. So none of us could communicate with one another outside of frantic hand gestures and furrowed facial expressions.

Pointing to the weapons trucks was all I needed to clarify our purpose for being there.

The trucks were parked out past the checkpoint blast walls. Kurdo nervously tugged at my jacket, begging me to stay behind for safety. His anxiety was understandable. Just a few months earlier, a large supply truck had tried to enter through a checkpoint and blew up as it was searched.

Of course I was anxious, but I did not intend to stand behind blast walls, shouting out orders to people, if that were even possible. I looked in the back of the trucks and dropped my head into my hands. There were at least a thousand weapons just tossed into the bed of the truck in a massive heap. I figured this haphazard arrangement was what was making the guards nervous, so we made our way back to the checkpoint.

The Georgians called for their chain of command, and ten minutes later a Georgian captain and a lieutenant showed up. The lieutenant was at least six-foot-four, spoke no English, and looked and sounded like Dolph Lundgren from *Rocky IV*. He wore a crisp uniform and sported a pair of sleek sunglasses.

Standing next to this giant was a Georgian captain of five-foot-four with workable English. He seemed competent, but he looked as if he were just pulled out of a duffle bag. His uniform was incomplete, his equipment unsnapped, his helmet band pulled away from his chin, and a cigarette dangled from his lips.

The Georgians were all new to the job, so the captain didn't

even know the source of the problem. He finally came to me and
said in a thick Russian accent, "All amu-nicion trooks mus goo too
Chackpont 2, ser." My mind flashed. *Checkpoint 2 was the same
place that truck exploded a few months ago.* Kurdo explained that
the drivers had come instead to this checkpoint because they were
terrified of being hijacked with the same result as the other truck.

In my most polite voice, I told the Georgian captain I worked
for the Iraqi chief of defense and begged his help *just this once.* He
nodded with his eyes closed, as if he were willing to help, but not
all that happy about doing it.

The little, rumpled captain then turned to Dolph and gave
a casual instruction. The lieutenant nodded with an intense gaze
then swung his radio off his back like a broad sword. He spoke into
the radio with a tone and volume that made it sound as if he were
ordering an airstrike on our position, *"Alpa ex-rey, alpa ex-rey, slokem
yak solum snowdney, glock snukem sleepney gope, jeneraley Iraqi mit,"*
he paused to look at my name tag, *"Mayore Waberi ... jeneraley
Iraqi mit, Mayore Wa-beri."*

(I paraphrase, with apologies to Russian-speaking people
everywhere.)

After some discussion and disagreements, approval was granted
for the trucks to be searched at that checkpoint and allowed to pass.
It was a small victory, and I really wondered what I had achieved.
Had I just taught Kurdo and the Georgians that rules were meant
to be broken?

While the trucks were being scanned, I hung out with the
drivers behind a blast wall. Through gestures and smiles, they tried
to explain how thirsty and hungry they were and showed me their
Iraqi money, as if I were a snack vendor; they had been too scared
to stop anywhere for any reason.

When their trucks cleared, I told them to follow me through
the city to the defense ministry. Out of ignorance or complete
disregard, they bolted out ahead of me as if someone had dropped

a green flag on race day. They drove like sixteen-year-olds on a go-cart track, passing each other on corners and driving their trucks, teetering with weapons, as hard as they could.

As we sped through the city, my head still throbbed from the fall, and the dried blood on my forehead stuck to the inner band of my Kevlar like glue. But I was fine. Everything was fine. And this perspective helped me separate the danger of the situation from the humor of the outcome.

If Nietzsche had had a better sense of humor, he would have said, "Anything that doesn't kill you makes you funnier."

✳ ✳ ✳

Joseph Heller never wrote another great comic novel after *Catch-22*. Maybe that's because he didn't have cancer.

Six years after my day as a gunrunner, I found myself in Rosemount, Minnesota, in December. Matthew, you had a swim meet, Kristin was already there, and I was running late. I texted Kristin for a reminder on the location. "Lakeville South High School." I Googled the directions, grabbed something to eat, then darted out the door.

Thirty minutes into the thirty-five-minute drive, the massive wad of bandages covering the deep incision in my abdomen sprang a leak, and I could feel warm bile and pancreatic fluid dripping down my belly and into my pants. (These fluids are caustic and were responsible for "eating" the hole in my abdomen since the surgery a year prior.)

Cursing myself for not having changed the bandages before I left, I reached over in the dark to the passenger seat for my "travel bag" of bandages, but nothing was there. I pictured them right where I left them at the back door.

Adjust fire!

I remembered there was a Target store in nearby Lakeville, so I altered course. I cursed myself while grabbing every fast-food napkin I could find in my glove box in an attempt to control the growing mess in my waistband. (Just to give you some perspective, I would go through about 24 four-by-four bandages per day. But on "heavy days"—yes, ladies, this guy can relate—it would be double that number. That day . . . was a *heavy* day.)

The idea of buying some diapers crossed my mind when I saw they sold only individually packaged bandages, ten to a box. And there were only two boxes left on the shelf. That would never carry me for the next four hours. (Yes, the "lady products" aisle is now part of my emergency response plan for future incidents, but I was still learning then.)

Disgusted with my circumstances, and feeling pressure to make it to Matthew's meet on time, I snatched the boxes from the shelf, made my way through checkout, and then ducked into the store bathroom. I lifted my shirt and just let the two-dozen, bright-yellow, bile-soaked napkins drop into the sink. Then I peeled off the mass of tape and soaked bandages and let that fall into the sink as well.

I needed something to wipe the acidic bile off my skin, so I went into a stall for some toilet paper, still holding my shirt up to my chin to keep it from getting any more soiled.

As I turned to go back to the sink, an employee walked in. His eyes got as big as saucers as he took in the scene:

Man standing in the middle of the bathroom with one hand holding a massive wad of toilet paper, his other hand holding his shirt up to his chin; standing next to a stinky, yellow, bandage-and-napkin-filled sink; sporting an exposed gut with a highly visible seventeen-inch-wide scar, a bullet-hole-looking open wound with yellow ooze coming out of it, and tubing with a big drainage bag hanging in full view, apparently full of shit.

I saw an imaginary cartoon bubble appear above his head with the words, "What kind of freak show we got goin' on in here?"

He awkwardly offered to help or get help, but I told him I had things under control. "It looks worse than it is . . . honest . . . I'm fine."

When I finally exited the bathroom, it was like hearing one of those record player needles screech off the vinyl. Every employee at those registers glanced my way as if I were a car crash on the freeway. My accident was tying up traffic. At Target.

The bandage debacle now had me running further behind schedule. As I pulled up to the school, I sighed with frustration; the place looked like an industrial complex, and there was no external signage. "Just come in the main entrance. You can't miss it," Kristin had said. "And hurry, his race is coming up."

I glanced up at a directional sign in the foyer with arrows on it—no mention of any swimming pool. There were kids *everywhere*. "Excuse me," I asked as one of them scurried past me. "Can you tell me where the swimming pool is?" He looked at me with a blank stare and said nothing. I pressed, "Are you *from* this school?" He finally mumbled in reply, "Uh, yeah . . . um, I don't think we have a swimming pool?"

I called Kristin back. "The people here tell me they don't have a swimming pool. They said their pool is at a place called Kenwood Middle School."

"Well," she said, "I don't know what to tell you. I saw the sign, and it said Lakeville South. Better hurry—you're going to miss Matthew."

It turned out to be at Kenwood.

I was incensed.

Matthew's race came and went, and as if on cue, my inadequate Target bandages began to leak again. I was partly mad at Kristin for what I thought were wrong directions, but I was madder at myself for being mad at her. I had no one to blame but myself, and I knew it.

I roared home, pissed at the world. Not only did I miss a race Matthew had prepared hard for, but stinky, warm bile continued to leak down into my pants, which were now soaked through to the crotch. It felt as if I were slowly peeing on myself, and there was nothing I could do about it. No more bandages. No more fast-food napkins.

Suddenly . . . lights. Red and blue, in my rearview mirror. *Think it can't get worse, Weber? Way to go. Dumbass.*

"License and registration, please," the state trooper said politely from out of view on the driver's side. I handed him my license.

Within a second, he asked, "Are you active duty military?" (I had Iraq War license plates and a dress uniform in the backseat.)

"Yes, sir."

He handed back my ID and stepped into full view. "Forget the registration. Do you know why I pulled you over?"

"Yes, sir," I said. "I was speeding . . . I know I was speeding." I used a tone that was humble but not pitiful. I had no excuse, and I wasn't going to offer one.

"Why you in such a hurry?" he asked.

"I've just got an awful mess here, and I suppose I just got in a hurry to get home," I answered.

"What's wrong?" he asked.

I laughed and said, "Well, this is going to sound shameless since I was speeding, but because you're asking . . . " I lifted my shirt to reveal my Frankenstein mess. "It's this."

His face looked like that employee's from Target. "Do you need some help? Can you still drive . . . can I get you somewhere?"

"I know it looks bad, but I'm honestly fine . . . it's just a mess, and I'm trying to get home."

He dispensed with the small talk. "Well, you take it easy, and just slow down for me, okay?"

"Yes, sir."

"And thank you for your service," he added.

✲ ✲ ✲

Not all tears are tears of sadness or despair. Sometimes they come from unbounded pride and joy, and I do believe if there is such a thing as a tonic for the soul, it is that feeling.

Matthew, you were a shy and quiet freshman, a personality you've carried in the extreme since birth, at least around your parents. Several months after my massive surgery in August 2010, you said you were trying out for a solo in the school choir. Kristin and I dismissed the idea, thinking you probably just meant a tryout for the choir itself.

After weeks of updates, you came home and yelled to me in the backyard, "Hey, Dad, I got the solo!" I went to Kristin and said, "He's serious. What the heck do you think is going on here? Can you see him singing a freakin' solo?"

"No," she said with a smile. "This should be interesting."

Of course we believed you were capable, but this spotlight-seeking was completely uncharacteristic.

We went to the choir concert with the expectation of seeing an overambitious freshman get an A for effort, but we were in for a surprise. Your voice boomed, you were in complete harmony with the piano, and we were enlightened.

A few months later, you sang again. We were better prepared this time but still in a state of disbelief. Looking at the program pamphlet, we learned you had earned a varsity letter and were one of three students voted by your peers as Most Valued Choir Member—two distinctions you hadn't mentioned to us. While we were attempting to process that information, the performance began.

The song was listed as "Tell My Father," which neither of us had heard before. You not only sang in tune, but with a conviction and emotion that was foreign to me until that moment.

"Tell my father that his son didn't run . . . or surrender. That I

bore his name with pride . . . as I tried . . . to remember . . . you
are judged by what you do, while passing through."

My eyes burst with tears as I tried to catch my breath. The
rest of the choir joined you, and the words continued to strip me
bare to the bone. The song was a ballad about an American Civil
War soldier, telling an unknown messenger to tell his father that
he wore his blue uniform—the same dress uniform I wear today—
with pride, that he bore the necessary sacrifice, that he had become
a man, and that his father should not cry for him.[11]

I could see you belting out the words with great emotion as you
glanced at us periodically out of the corner of your eye.

Did you really understand the full meaning behind the song?
Your solo contained words and ideas you had heard from me on
countless occasions, particularly since my diagnosis—to be strong
and courageous in the face of the unknown, and that you are judged
by your actions in this life. And of course you knew my passion for
soldiering, but did you also remember my intense interest in the
American Civil War? Or was the theme just coincidental? You were
always quiet with us about your emotions and thoughts, particularly with the cancer, and I desperately wanted to believe you were
communicating directly to me through this song.

"Tell him we will meet again . . . where the angels learn to fly.
Tell him we will meet as men, for with honor . . . did I die."

It was the last song of the concert. I didn't know what to expect
from you as you quietly approached me with a stoic look on your
face. I tried to keep it together as I reached out to you, without
saying a word, and quickly pulled you tight into my chest as the
tears uncontrollably filled my eyes again. I felt your body softly
jostle a bit in my arms as you gently cried, squeezed me just a little

---

11. Matthew's performance can be viewed at www.tellmysons.com.

tighter, and said, "I love you, Dad."

I chuckled out of embarrassment. I rarely heard those words and had never heard them spoken with such emotion. They made my throat tighten more. I tried to lighten the moment, for both our sakes. "My God, it sounded like you were singing to me, buddy."

"I was, Dad," you said.

★ ★ ★

Countless readers of my online journal have apologized for laughing while they've had tears in their eyes over the past two years. But I think this is actually the sweet spot MacArthur was talking about.

I propose to you that there is a time and a place for crying and laughing. And figuring out how to cry and laugh at hardship or death is a skill worth honing into a fine art when you're young.

Have you ever noticed how laughing babies never fail to bring us a smile and a warm feeling, no matter how we feel? Endorphins don't just happen; you have to find a laughter trigger.

Do you boys remember the times I got you to laugh when you were sad or mad? I'd get you to crack, but you tried like hell to keep that smile or laugh from coming through. You refused it.

We all seem to find it much easier to let ourselves cry. See what happens when you let yourself laugh.

Many times in a good life, you'll laugh until you cry. And many other times, you'll cry until you laugh. In the end, laughing and crying are more like cousins than strangers. They're how honest human beings respond to a life they allow themselves to love, and my hope is that you have plenty of tears in your lives—of all kinds.

CHAPTER EIGHT

... TO DISCOVER THE SENSE OF WONDER, THE
UNFAILING HOPE OF WHAT IS NEXT, AND THE JOY
AND INSPIRATION OF LIFE.

November 2010

Just three months after my original diagnosis and life-altering surgery, I was honored at a Minnesota Vikings football game in front
of sixty-four thousand fans. I stood on that field in my army dress
uniform, looking fairly pathetic—and feeling even worse.

Under my uniform, I was a train wreck. I was barely able to
stand in my emaciated 130-pound frame.

What on earth was I doing at this grand-scale pity party?

The announcer briefly outlined my service in the army and said
I was being honored as their Hometown Hero. Scattered applause
followed.

Then he explained that I had been preparing for another
combat tour that summer, handpicked by General Petraeus to serve

with him in Afghanistan, but within weeks had been diagnosed with stage IV cancer. The crowd went silent.

He went on to describe my perseverance and attitude since being diagnosed, introduced my wife and children, and then announced my name as if he were introducing a gladiator in the Roman Colosseum.

Those sixty-four thousand fans jumped to their feet and exploded with applause. I could clearly see the faces of men and women wiping tears from their eyes in front of me. The announcer then had to yell over the crowd that they were going to promote me to lieutenant colonel.

In the video of the event, the applause was so deafening that the announcer just stopped speaking.[12]

When the game was over, Noah (then ten years old) commented, "Dad, you looked like you were going to cry the whole time. Why were you so sad?"

"Because having cancer doesn't make me a hero, and I just wouldn't be standing out there without it."

It was Chaplain John Morris, our state chaplain and a good friend, who helped convince me I needed to change my thinking about the Vikings game and what my story meant to other people. He helped me realize that the tribute wasn't much different than fourth down in a clutch situation in a big football game.

The passion of the crowd wasn't necessarily focused on what I had achieved, but in the unfailing hope—their unfailing hope—of what was still possible to overcome.

The message from the crowd during that "fourth-down play," as I have come to interpret it, wasn't pity or sorrow, but hope—and love of another human being: "*That* is a guy I want to see fight and win!"

✯ ✯ ✯

---

12. The tribute can be seen at www.tellmysons.com.

May 2012

Nineteen months after standing on that football field, I was much worse for wear but able and willing to acknowledge an incredible sense of wonder at still being alive and an unexpected discovery of joy and inspiration for life.

My feeding tube had been removed, I had just finished penning a first-ever strategic communication plan for the Minnesota National Guard, and all my garden's flowers were in full bloom.

I still had a visible "bullet hole" in my abdomen and a catheter running through my ribs and liver, but the pain and nuisance had long become tolerable. I even got used to the idea of putting up with one or two bouts of sepsis per month, as my body seemed capable of fighting back so effectively in the thirty episodes I had experienced so far.

Then on Memorial Day, some trouble with the bullet hole prompted me to visit the hospital. Dr. Ehrenwald ("Oscar") ran a quick X-ray to gain some perspective on the size of the hole, and then we retired to his office to check it out.

When the image of my abdomen appeared on the screen, my internal organs were as immediately familiar to me as the features on my own face. Forget the bullet hole. What I noticed instead was that the biggest tumor in my liver—the one that had been as large as a silver dollar—was now twice as big. And two of the other fifteen tumors were clearly "awake" again.

Some people get ten years; others get less than one, I remembered. The news felt as devastating as my initial diagnosis.

I immediately started a new chemo treatment, but it crashed on takeoff. My skin and eyes turned yellow, my body started itching, my urine turned tea colored, I was frequently short of breath, and I felt tired all the time—all telltale signs of a liver in severe distress. They even had to stick a catheter through my back and drain a liter of fluid off my right lung again.

I envisioned my entire fighting position being overrun and surrounded, just as it had been in the fall of 2010. Gone was the desire to boldly declare war. As in real combat, the harsh reality of battle had tempered my approach.

At work, I decided to permanently hand off my proverbial saber and guidon to my relief. *Soldiers and officers come and go*, we say, *the army lives on.* Leaving the army is a day that comes for every soldier; I just selfishly wished it were more on my terms.

Was this quitting? I'll let you in on a little secret: the army doesn't quit or retreat—*ever.* We've come up with our own language to cheat the system a bit. We "consolidate," we "reorganize," we "conduct retrograde operations," but we *never* "quit" or "retreat." So what's the difference between retrograde operations and retreating? *Attitude.* Or as I like to call it, *the middle finger.*

I think if there had been an army battalion aboard the Titanic, I would have been fully and unapologetically engaged in ordering the deck chairs to be rearranged when all other options ran out. That's not denial, and it's *not* positive thinking. I know the ship is going down, and my attitude might actually be crappy. I would just rather do *something*, because the truth is, I no longer know how to do nothing.

✯ ✯ ✯

June 2012

Boys, my failing health did not bring you to my side for a heart-to-heart chat now any more than it had at the beginning. In fact, you were all fairly dismissive about the news. Kristin and I shared a brief moment of tears, but she was just as quick to declare that I was so stubborn, I would probably be the first human to live without a liver. And you all seemed to share her contempt for the idea that anything could bring me down.

But it will.

We hadn't talked about the "what ifs" in any serious detail since the fall of 2010. Now the time had come, and you were all resistant. Matthew, because you were older, you were my primary focus, and I searched for a way to get at the subject.

When the army put me on full medical leave June 1, I had already been slated to speak at the Minnesota History Center in celebration of the Army's 237th birthday on June 14. I searched for army themes I could carry. Sacrifice? Honor? Determination? Humility?

Tell him that I wore the blue, proud and true, through the fire. Tell my father so he'll know ... I love him so.

A duet.

The idea hit me so fast and hard, I was crying over my keyboard before I could complete the thought. *Music.* This was one of the ways you communicated, Matthew.

Fighting and surviving a civil war. Dying. The Army Blue dress uniform. Carrying a message. Never quitting. Love. Nearly every word *spoke to me, to you, to all of us in this terrible moment in our lives.* And a perfect tribute to the army, to boot. (The fact it was also Father's Day was a happy coincidence.)

When you enthusiastically agreed to sing this emotionally explosive song with your dying father in front of an audience of strangers, I knew at the very least we shared the "crazy" gene.[13]

When that performance was done, the idea for *Tell My Sons . . .* was born. As difficult as it was for us to talk about life now, I believed you would be curious in the future, and this book would be the next best thing to my side of the conversation.

✷ ✷ ✷

July 2012

I started my fourth chemo trial—a kidney cancer treatment—in

---

13. The speech and the performance can be seen at www.tellmysons.com.

mid-July. That same week, I received a call from General Dempsey's office, which just happened to be the same week he and I received our respective cancer diagnoses two years prior. Dempsey had not only beaten his throat cancer but had since been elevated to the most senior position in the US Army, and within months of that promotion had been selected by President Obama to serve as the most senior officer in the entire US Armed Forces as the eighteenth chairman of the Joint Chiefs of Staff.

If his travel plans allowed it, he and his wife, Deanie, wanted to come to Minnesota to honor me and Kristin for our service in the army. By the time August 16 rolled around, General Jack Vessey, the tenth chairman of the Joint Chiefs of Staff, had decided to join us.

Hearing Dempsey speak about our work together and his personal assessment of my character in front of 350 of my friends and family made me feel as if I were witnessing my own eulogy.

> *It's now Lieutenant Colonel Weber educating General Dempsey... that the greatest value of a life is to spend it for something that lives after it. That in the end you become what you are through the causes to which you attach yourself - and that you've made your own along the way. And that in many ways, it can be a far higher ideal in life to live an ordinary life in an extraordinary way. I'll always remember those lessons from Mark Weber. That's what [he] taught me.[14]*

General Pace, the sixteenth chairman of the Joint Chiefs of Staff, couldn't be there in person, but he sent a message. In summarizing what he thought of my work and my fight, he reached back to our little joke, "To borrow from a near famous quote: Damn. He's good."

---

14. General Dempsey's remarks at the ceremony and also my remarks can be seen at www. tellmysons.com.

David Petraeus, now the director of the CIA (and a frequent e-mail pen pal), also sent along a note, "I know that you've been fighting a courageous personal battle since I almost had you on a plane to Afghanistan two years ago, and I truly have been inspired by your bravery and grit."

Of course, I was flattered by such affirmation from these titans of my profession, but I also heard a charge of responsibility to continue to do what I had done all my life in the army—until the day I die.

Which was fine with me.

As the former Navy Seal Eric Greitens would say, the mission *does* continue. And as my friends in Outward Bound would say, as long as a ship is seaworthy, the Blue Peter nautical flag, indicating the vessel is "outward bound," should always be flown.

Chaplain Morris summarized the sentiment as he continued to encourage me to share this book with the public:

We are bombarded daily by truly bad news—war, rumors of war, accidents, murders, and on and on. Couple that with the challenges that each human being faces, and it's no wonder that most of us are in need of inspiration. The problem is that the most inspirational people in our midst rarely share their life story. They simply work their way through each day, doing what they do best—facing life head on with determination, endurance and courage. We need those people to share their stories so we can draw inspiration from them for the living of our lives. You have one of those stories and you should share it.

✯ ✯ ✯

November 2012

Everyone's clock is ticking. But my clock, we can hear. What will tomorrow bring for us?

If MacArthur were alive today, I think he would agree with me that if you are able to draw from the morals in the preceding chapters, you will naturally and graciously receive the gifts of this *chapter: a sense of wonder, the unfailing hope of what is next, and the joy and inspiration of life.*

I have, and I'm not done seeking out and discovering. I'm not done asking questions. I'm not done learning. Because I am still alive.

I propose to you that pain and suffering—self-inflicted or otherwise—is not merely a rude interruption of your journey, but one of the very purposes of the journey. The Bufords of your life aren't something to ignore or eliminate (if that were even possible). They are meant to be confronted with the very best effort you can give for as long as you are able. Your bravery, your honesty, your pride and humility, your appetite for adventure, your love for others, your imagination, your wisdom, your seriousness and emotional expression—these are brought to bear not by the sweet and easy moments of your life, though you should savor those too, but in confrontation with your Bufords.

If I'm truly and finally proud of anything in my life, it is that I lived it in constant striving, continuous searching, and willing struggle, while conducting as honest an exploration of this world as I knew how to do.

If you wonder whether you'll live your life this way, think about this: Where would you be today if you accepted the wisdom you had at age ten? Should you accept the wisdom life has granted you at age twenty or thirty or forty? Or will you continue to ask questions and seek to broaden your understanding of yourself and the world around you? I already know you well enough to have a pretty good idea of what you'll do.

I've shared with you how these morals and ideas have guided me, and I've made some proposals to you.

But maybe it's most important for you to know this:

Knowing you, knowing each of you—Matthew, Joshua, Noah—I have complete faith that you'll *figure it out.*

I love you so.

EPILOGUE
"How Are You Doing?"

Imagine loading your spouse and kids into the family car for a day-trip across town. Instead of driving the highways, you're going to take a narrow ATV trail—*a route you've never even seen before.* The only catch is that once you start for the day, *and you must,* you can try to slow down, but you won't be able to stop.

Now blindfold your spouse and kids.

Repeat this drive every single day until you die.

This is what life has been like for me, Kristin, Matthew, Joshua, and Noah. As the driver, I can see what's in front of me once we start each day. I can feel the gas, clutch, brake, and steering wheel as we crash into obstacles and careen through rough turns, small jumps, and steep drops and climbs. It's a rough ride for all of us, but at least I can see where I'm headed and have some sense of control. We'll make this harrowing drive until I die and my journey will be over for good.

Kristin and our boys can obviously see more than a blindfold would allow, but they have no control over what happens, aside from offering the same thing friends and family are desperately saying to all of us over the walkie-talkie speakers piped through our radio: encouragement and advice about how to drive and occasional outbursts of sadness or anger at the inevitable setbacks of the trip.

My boys will lose a father at an age when most people lose a grandfather.

And Kristin? How can words possibly describe the pain and loss of a love tempered by the book you've just read? Or practically speaking, the loss of the disciplinarian to our boys and primary source of income for our family? Sadness and fear do not *begin* to describe the feelings.

"How are you doing?" is the most common question we've heard since we started this journey. In fact, journalist David Murray, with whom I collaborated on this book, made an observation about that question one month into our work. In describing the first time he met us all in Chicago, he observed:

> *When I was with your family for those two hours in Chicago, I felt like I was looking into a window of pain verging on madness, in all of you—you, the kids, Kristin. What came to mind was a frank acknowledgment on my part of the uncertainty, the fear, and the anger you must still feel . . . I'd like you to acknowledge that even the goriest and most gut-wrenching parts of the book doesn't quite portray the near madness, the insane sadness, the utter fear and confusion . . . the disordering and swirling reality of the situation.*

The problem for me is that I don't think it's possible to fully capture inside a few pages the raw and disorderly experience David and so many others would like to know.[15]

What is written here is meant to give you some sense of how we're tackling our cancer fight. But it does require something on your part as the reader. You have to set aside your own imagination about what you think it *must* be like and trust that what I am telling you *is* what it is like. Because I cannot compete with imagination.

---

15. The closest I can come to such description is my CaringBridge journal— www.caringbridge.org/visit/markmweber.

Everyone in our family has handled things slightly differently, which is offered here as observation rather than a judgment of what's good or bad, or what works or doesn't work.

Joshua processes his emotions and thoughts inside and doesn't share them with many people. He's always right in the moment and not often one step further. If he had a credo at this age it might be, "I'll cross that bridge when I get there."

One morning at about 6:00 a.m., he came downstairs while I was having my coffee and asked to sit with me in my favorite La-Z-Boy—the one we've had since *Matthew* was a baby. He lay sideways in my arms, and I cradled him and snuggled in close, just as we have every few weeks or so since he was little.

We rocked back and forth while I spoke my heart about the impact cancer was going to have, trying to give him a sense of how much he meant to me and how I was feeling. I was misty eyed as I asked him how he was feeling. I felt him jostling in my arms, as if he were crying. But when I looked down into his face, I saw he was giggling! It actually made me a bit upset.

"Joshua! How can you laugh about such a thing? This is serious."

He seemed embarrassed but kept on giggling as he replied, "Your *breath* stinks, Dad."

Noah is very different. He wears his emotions on his sleeve, and he speaks his mind and asks questions not long after a thought has been formed. His most pressing question was what would happen when I was gone. Will we have to sell the house? Change schools?

Just a few months ago, when my third chemo treatment failed, he asked Kristin in a deadpan, "Will I get a stepdad?" (Kristin replied, "No, we'll get another cat. I'm going to be a cat lady." And this answer seems to satisfy him, though I'm not sure what it says about me!)

To be honest, such experiences, combined with others shared in the book, did not encourage me at all about "how they were doing." So it came as some surprise when their school social worker, Jim Ciemny, wrote to me out of the blue, asking for my permission to let Joshua and Noah help another student.

Help? *My boys?*

Jim wrote, "I have witnessed some pretty amazing stuff with your children, and I am profoundly changed because of it . . . there is an agreement of sorts, or pact if you will, between the two. They both agree that Noah is more 'hands on and emotional,' while Josh is comfortable with being 'perimeter support and more quiet,' to use their words. Their ability to communicate, assign roles, and strategize is pretty amazing and advanced for their age. Simply put, it is empathy in motion."

Jim has been working in his field for twenty years and spent half of his career working with troubled youth and broken families. He went on to explain there was a third grader whose father was a soldier who had been deployed for most of the past two years. The child was beginning to express intense stress (unconscious self-mutilation), anxiety, frustration, and a reduced ability to focus on academics. While brainstorming about how to best support the boy, multiple teachers and specialists suggested Joshua and Noah as potential mentors.

I was more than a little concerned. I could only *imagine* Joshua and Noah were already carrying enough heavy rocks with a dad and two grandparents fighting cancer. Still, in my own profession, I had personally experienced how helping others had actually *lifted* personal burdens, so I agreed.

The boys were elated.

"And oh boy did they help," Jim later wrote. Joshua and Noah met with the young boy every week. "Surprisingly," Jim said, "Joshua was the most verbal, assuring, and comforting role model for this child. He'd ask gentle questions and share his thoughts. Noah did as well, but his effort was more expected given his outspoken nature. It seemed mutually therapeutic for all involved.

By the end of the school year the third grader was stable, and he routinely sought out your children *more than me* when he needed to be heard and affirmed. Talk about reciprocal fellowship!"

For two years, Jim said he saw the full range of emotions—sorrow, profound grief, tears, humor, sarcasm, silence, and joy. All of which was expected and normal, in his view. "They *do* complain, but it always comes back to you and Kristin and how much they feel loved."

Jim closed his note telling us Joshua and Noah reflected two themes every time he saw them, and he just had to believe we emulated in our home: "Know where you started, where you are, and where you want to be; and don't *ever* give up."

✯ ✯ ✯

Matthew is in a category by himself. As a teenager, he's struggling with hormones, testy emotions, girlfriends, the rigors of succeeding and failing in sport, and high school life in general. Who's to say what emotion comes from where? He certainly can't tell, and he can't explain exactly what he feels or thinks about it all, so I don't think the answer can be known.

Rather than focusing on why the emotions are there or what generates them, I offered that it might matter more to focus on what to do about it. Because he couldn't control what he felt or when he felt it, perhaps it was best to work on things within his control—*behavior and environment.*

On one particularly rough day, we sat together on the couch and he had a good, long cry. "Nothing is going right; everything is going wrong. It sucks!" he finally said with anger and tears in his eyes.

He doesn't like to talk about what life will be like without a dad, and he has always resisted talks with me or others about it. On that day, I insisted. He and I sat at the kitchen table while Kristin cleaned up after dinner.

I grabbed a glass of water, filled it halfway up, and set it in front
of him. "This glass of water represents your life," I offered. "We all
have a pretty easy time of describing this part," I said as I pointed
to the empty half of the glass. "That's fine, and we need to do that
to keep our grip on reality and stay humble. But sometimes we have
to work a little harder to figure out what's in this part of the glass
here," and I pointed to the water. "What's the water in your life?"
I asked him.

He sat there thinking for several minutes, speechless. "Well,
I'm not sick," he finally said.

I chuckled. "Well, now we know what you're not. Let's focus on
what you *are*. Focus on what you have, not what you don't have."

He continued to look at the table in front of him, his face
contorted in discomfort. Nothing.

"Let's start with something really close to you," I offered. "Your
mom and dad—give us a rating."

"Well," he said, "you don't abuse me or treat me poorly." Again,
I reiterated the need to focus on what he has, not what he doesn't
have. Then he started getting it as he rattled off what we do for him
and how we show our love and care for him, even when we're upset
with his behavior.

"How about your girlfriend?" I asked. "She's smart, pretty,
and two grades ahead of you, but she would rather have you as a
boyfriend than any of the boys in her class. What do you think that
says about you?"

He shrugged his shoulders and said he never really thought
about it that way.

"You try now," I said. Still, he sat there dumbfounded. After a
few minutes of silence, I asked, "What about your guitar?"

His head shot up. Yes. He was damned good at playing the
guitar. He had worked hard to get there, and he didn't need to be
Jimi Hendrix to relish some pride in his abilities.

"How about your singing or the dedication and passion you

put into swimming?" I asked.

"Yeah, but I'm not good enough to keep up with the older boys," he responded.

I tapped on the empty half of the glass. "Yes, it's important to know what you don't yet possess and need to work at, but we want to focus here," I shifted my finger, "on the water, on the part where there is *something*."

He finally acknowledged that although he wasn't where he wanted to be in swimming, he really had come a long way. In fact, he could see this logic in just about everything he did, from riding a bike to handwriting.

The whole discussion took twenty-five minutes. As we finished, he shifted in his seat, looked me in the eyes, and said with an apparent sadness, "This is hard." *Yes. It is. But you get better at it the more you practice.*

✳ ✳ ✳

Kristin, of course, is as close to the details and the roller coaster drama as I am. Her modesty means getting her to talk about life's blessings is as difficult as prying it from Matthew. In all of her life, it's always been good enough to just live in the day, with her gut instincts and, privately, without much worry for tomorrow.

From religion to politics to the meaning of life, her thoughts are locked up tighter than Fort Knox. Not even my deployments would pry her tongue. She's never had a problem acknowledging hardships and expressing sadness or anger with her own Bufords, but she's always been content to distract herself with a few small hobbies, with the housework that needs to be done, or with the three sons she enjoys nurturing.

But with my cancer at age thirty-eight? And both parents with cancer in their early sixties? Everything about this experience has forced her to open the locks on her vault. She's private, but she's not a recluse, so it's much harder to maintain the balance she desires with how much and when to share.

"Is it okay for me to laugh or have fun when my husband is dying of cancer?" she says through tears that turn a heart inside out. "I feel guilty. I should be here with you." It doesn't matter what I tell her or what her friends say. Her character tells her it's wrong, and she abides.

She knows life isn't fair, and she knows she's not alone or unique in her hardship, but the anger and frustration still pound at her door every day.

Drainage bags, open sores, dangling medical implants, and a twenty-four-hour shit-smell put one hell of a damper on life as you might imagine it for a husband and wife at age forty. I'm not an invalid by a long shot, and I am physically capable in every conceivable way, but our lives are routinely punctuated by periods of complete misery that carry a dramatic impact.

These conditions have *redefined the meaning of love, affection, and commitment* for both of us virtually overnight. They have propelled us into a relationship more often seen at age seventy than forty. Considering the foundation we had going into cancer, our transition has been relatively smooth, but it has not been without struggle. The same prescription we've tried to employ for eighteen years still seems to apply—*communicate, and if you must fight, fight fair and be gracious in the makeup.*

Nothing brings me to tears faster than the firm belief that Kristin will carry the vast majority of the *near madness, the insane sadness, the utter fear and confusion, and the disordering and swirling reality of the situation* David spoke of in his question.

To use Kristin's words: "Yes, life is unfair, but it seems just a little more so knowing that you're going to lose your best friend who is seemingly unfazed by the trials of life, and a soul mate who you just know brings out the very best in you—*even as he pisses you off every now and again.*"

★ ★ ★

What people really seem to want to know is, *what's it like to die in slow motion . . . to actually see your own death approaching?*

Today? And speaking only for myself? It sucks. It's beautiful. It's terrifying. It's pure torture. It's pure joy. And it feels a little irresponsible (because I know I'm going to leave my family for something I know will be better).

If you believe that life owes us nothing and we owe it everything; that life is all about the *fullest* possible experience of the ride, good and bad; and that death is part of life—then there is a strange peace and comforting resolution to seeing it all unfold in front of you, even as it scares the hell out of you to know you're leaving your family in a lurch.

We all know, or have at least heard, that Death is supposed to come to us like a thief in the night. I caught Death trying to break in, and I've somehow managed to kick him in the teeth—for two years. With anger, happiness, and sadness welling up inside of me as I write this, *can you imagine how good that makes me feel as a soldier or in light of what you've read about my life?*

Death is going to get in, but I know right where he's at. Considering the fact that Death is coming for all of us, the ability to see him coming and make it happen on my terms has to be the next best thing to living a long life.

I've experienced half a dozen curtain calls and am actually beginning to feel a little guilty for not meeting expectations. My funeral is going to be downright anticlimactic.

I say all of this with great humility, because every once in a while, I do reach down and grab hold of the electrified rail that is my reality from day to day and week to week.

Kristin and I were once discussing some routine tidbit on life, and she suddenly interrupted me, almost as if she were irritated by me poking fun at death. "Don't you get angry or frustrated with all of this? Nothing ever seems to faze you with this stuff."

The fact is, I do get angry. For example, I believe attitude and prayer are important, but I do get upset when people insist these are the causes and the cures for cancer.

And it's not true that nothing fazes me. A lot of shit fazes me. In each of the dozen or so times I've been flat on my ass for days on end—believe me, I was fazed.

So then what? That's my question about getting angry or fazed. The answer for me, for most of my adult life, has been just a few adapted lines from the Serenity Prayer I desperately try to practice: *Accept the things I cannot change, change the things that I can, and seek out information and perspective from others* (wisdom) *so I can tell the difference between the two.*

If I could, I would further edit the Serenity Prayer and add, "And later on, when you gain more wisdom, revisit the things you thought you couldn't change and try again."

I experience fear as well, but more so for what's going to happen to my family when I'm gone, not about what's coming for me. My faith tells me where I'm going. I'm not eager to leave, but I'm very excited to see what's on "the other side" of life.

My family cries, we yell, we laugh, and we *try* to talk about what all of this will ultimately mean for them. Mostly we focus on living the life we have and focusing on what we can do when things don't go as we want. On this last score, I am far more aggressive in providing authoritative leadership within my family and much less patient in accepting excuses.

If any of this—the stories to my boys or this epilogue to you— sounds like a prescription for how to deal with shitty things in your life, let me be *really* clear in declaring with great conviction that it's all an experiment in my view. And it's all easier said than done. All I know is that as long as I have been able, I have tried.

So if you cross paths with them in your life, I hope you'll *tell my sons* (or your sons or daughters) to pursue the morals in this story for as long as *they* are able.

Author's Note
and
Acknowledgements

I'm mildly allergic to overt displays of spirituality (I worry that they embarrass God), but I need to make an exception here, because to proceed without first acknowledging God's inspiration in my life wouldn't be right. I am thankful to God for inspiring me not just to be good, but to *be good for something;* and for his having enough faith in me to let me live life just as it seems he *must* have intended—*imperfectly.* The true wonder of this existence is that he has not tried to live my life for me nor relieved me of the experiences that have made me who and what I am.

I am proud of the life I have lived, but when people call me a "hero" or tell me how lucky my boys are to have me as a father, I look to my right and see my wife and closest friend, Kristin, and I am humbled. *She* is the hero because *she* is the reason I have been able to be the soldier, father, and man I am. In the case of this book, I got the "bonus plan," because despite the fact that cancer is stealing away my remaining time with her, she supports my efforts with love and care.

To my parents, Dennis and Illean. I'm sorry for being such a pain-in-the-ass child, but I hope I made up for it as a man. Thank you for the solid foundation and for always letting me be me.

Tell My Sons . . . was born out of the persistence and determination of Chaplain John Morris. Well over a year ago, I started combing through my twenty-plus years of journal entries and e-mails to collect some important stories I could share with my sons. John is the one who convinced me to produce a version I could share outside our four walls—with other sons and fathers and mothers and daughters.

My thanks to writer Jay Heinrichs, who was the first to help me wrestle with several approaches to writing the book and then encouraged me to write each story directly to Matthew, Joshua, and Noah.

When I wrote to David Murray on June 21, 2012, about collaborating on this book, his reply was a polite, "I probably ain't the guy for this." But the more we spoke, the more I knew he was *precisely* the right guy for this. Exactly one month later, he agreed to our partnership.

When he asked me what the timeline was, I told him a Christmas gift was my goal, which meant we needed to be done with a draft by the end of September—*just two months away.* He replied he didn't think that would be possible, but "I'm betting that you're just the kind of guy who will prove me wrong."

David *listened*, observed the common threads in my life, and then aggressively helped me find an approach I never would have found on my own. His candor, humor, objectivity, empathy, and keen eyes helped me transform my stories into My Story.

I owe an astonishing debt of gratitude to a number of people who helped me with this project. Kerri Alexander, Mitch Albom's copy editor, offered to copyedit this book and then insisted on doing it for free. Jim Kosmo, my literary agent, has provided counsel and friendship every step of the way. Tom Kerber and Amy Quale at Beaver's Pond Press treated me like royalty and made the business end of this project about as painless as I could ever have hoped for. And Paul Engleman provided an additional review and edit that helped this book along in a hundred little ways. To Shel Danielson and Scott Thomsen at Holton House Audio, and Whynn Grothem at Tri-Audio Productions, for their invaluable and generous help with the audiobook.

Drs. Timothy Sielaff, Eduardo Ehrenwald ("Oscar"), Subbarao Inampudi ("Felix"), John Seng, and, most notably, nurse practitioner Marie Kramer were more than just my medical team. They have been like family. Their ability to work together is how a fifth diagnosis became the *correct* diagnosis, so their gift to me has been the last two years of my life.

To the fifty-nine men and women who have received a 1971 silver dollar from me over the past eighteen years (you know who you are)—thank you for making me the person I am. Three mentors in particular deserve special mention, as they have been fathers to me during my *entire* time in the army: Colonel Terry Clemons, Command Sergeant Major Jim Barrett, and Colonel David Treuting. Aside from these three men, there's no way I can list more of you without inadvertently missing one of you. You simply *must* know who you are.

I've mostly used real names in this book. John Booth, Dennis Bryer, Ben Kramer, Avery James, and Mike Burns are all pseudonyms, so if one of their stories seems to be referring to you, it's either paranoia or wishful thinking.

My thanks to Major General Richard Nash, for granting me permission to write this book while still serving on active duty. Since I have decided to use my rank to identify myself as author, I'm obligated to express that the views presented in this book are mine and do not necessarily represent the views of Department of Defense.

In October 2010, several hundred family members and friends from across the country, as well as hundreds of soldiers and every senior leader in the Minnesota National Guard, gathered together to hold the *Operation True Grit* benefit for my family. I was reluctant to accept help we didn't *need*, and I didn't know what the hell I was going to do with all that generosity.

This book is part of the answer: the benefit raised nearly the exact amount of money needed to publish this book on my terms.

That generosity is also empowering us to take *Operation True Grit* and pay it forward. Kristin and I are going to use at least half of the proceeds of any money we make on this book to help other parents' sons and daughters overcome their hardships so they may live, as I hope my sons will, rich and productive and loving lives.

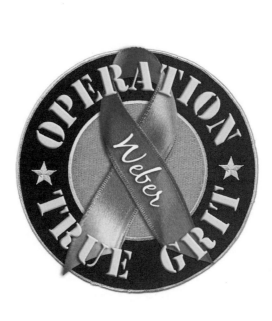